THE 2

Andrea Adams

Table of Contents

Part I

Chapter 1: Introduction

Today, many Americans are suffering from chronic diseases such as obesity and diabetes. In most cases, these diseases are a direct result of the kind of food we eat. The standard diet for a typical American contains excessive amounts of carbohydrates and proteins. Such a diet is not good for your health since it leads to the development of problems like insulin and leptin resistance. As a result, you end up gaining excess weight, developing inflammation, and putting yourself at risk of cellular damage.

To avoid these problems, you should make significant changes to your diet. One of the best ways of doing this is to induce a state of nutritional ketosis in your body. This is a state where your body uses stored fats as the primary source of energy, instead of using sugars. To get your body in this state, you have to follow a keto diet. But what exactly is a keto diet?

As someone who is conscious about your health and what you eat, you have probably heard about keto cleansing and the keto diet, also known as the ketogenic diet. The keto diet is a low-carb, high-fat diet that is popular among athletes and average folk alike. The keto diet is not new. It has been around for over a century. It was very popular in the 1920s and 1930s, but its use gradually faded in the 1940s. However, the keto diet has seen a resurgence in popularity recently as a specialized diet that has several health benefits.

This book will teach you everything you need to know about a keto diet. It will also give you a meal plan – complete with a variety of recipes to choose from – that will help you achieve a keto cleanse in 28 days.

Benefits Of Keto Cleansing

Undergoing ketogenic cleansing has several benefits for people who would like to improve their health, rapidly lose weight, or recover from chronic ailments.

Some of the Main Benefits of the Keto Diet Are:

Weight loss: If you are trying to shed some weight, undergoing keto cleansing is one of the best ways to do it since ketosis burns the stored fat and converts it into energy. Scientific studies have shown that a keto diet has far better weight loss results than low-fat and higher-carb diets.

Anti-inflammation: The human body can derive energy from sugar or fat. While the body uses sugar as the primary source of energy, fat is preferred in the keto diet because it is healthier and cleaner. Converting fat to energy produces fewer secondary free radicals and reactive oxygen species (ROS). By getting removing sugar from your diet, you decrease your chances of developing chronic inflammation.

Decreased risk of cancer: According to research by the University of South Florida, a keto diet can help lower the risk of getting cancer. All the cells in the body typically use glucose as a source of fuel. However, unlike normal body cells, cancerous cells are not metabolically flexible, which means that they cannot switch to using ketones as a source of energy. Once your body starts using ketones as the primary source of energy, the cancerous cells will starve to death.

Increased muscle mass: The structure of ketones is similar to that of branched-chain amino acids, which are essential for building muscle mass. When your body produces ketones, it frees up these amino acids to be used to increase muscle mass. This is why the keto diet is a favorite for athletes.

Increased energy and normalized hunger: Fat is a better and more reliable source of energy for the body. By converting fats to energy, your body feels more energized during the day. Fats are also more satisfying and keep the body in a satiated state for longer. This keeps hunger pangs at bay and makes you feel full and satisfied after eating.

Control blood sugar: By undergoing keto cleansing, you can control your blood sugar levels because you consume fewer carbs for the body to break down into sugars.

Studies have shown that a keto diet is an effective way of preventing and managing diabetes.

Lower insulin levels: When you consume carbs, the body breaks them down into sugars, causing a rise in your blood sugar levels. This in turn leads to production of more insulin. If this goes on for some time, you might develop insulin resistance, which can quickly progress to type 2 diabetes if unchecked. By limiting your intake of carbs through keto cleansing, you can reduce your risk of developing type 2 diabetes.

Better mental focus: Many people undergo keto cleansing specifically to increase their mental performance. Ketones are a better source of fuel for the brain compared to glucose. By keeping your carb intake low, you avoid spikes in blood sugar levels. This helps improve your focus and concentration.

Chapter 2: The Six Pillars Of Keto Diet Success
#1: Understanding The Nutrition

As was mentioned in the introduction, a keto diet is focused on minimizing the intake of carbs. Because of this, the keto diet is sometimes referred to as a low-carb diet or a low-carb, high-fat (LCHF) diet.

Normally, when you consume something that has a high carb content, two things happen within your body. The carbs are broken down into glucose, which is the easiest molecule that the body can use as a source of energy. The body will also produce insulin to help process the glucose.

Since your body uses the glucose as the primary source of energy, your fats have no immediate use and therefore the body stores them. This is what happens when you are on a normal, high-carb diet. However, when you decrease your intake of carbs through the keto diet, your body goes into a state known as ketosis. This is a natural state that the body uses to help us survive when there's low food intake. In this state, the body breaks down fats in the liver to produce ketones, which are then used as a source of energy.

The end goal of keto cleansing is to get your body into this metabolic state. However, instead of using starvation to do this, the keto diet achieves ketosis by depriving the body of carbohydrates. Since the body is highly adaptive, once you overload it with fats and deprive it of carbs, it will switch to using ketones as the primary source of energy.

Since the aim of keto cleansing is to reduce your intake of carbs, you should avoid grains such as rice, cereal, and wheat, sugars such as honey and maple syrup, fruits such as oranges, bananas, and apples and tubers such as potatoes and yams. Instead, you should increase your intake of meats, leafy greens, above ground vegetables, high-fat dairy, avocados and berries, nuts and seeds, low-carb sweeteners and other fats, such as coconut oil, saturated fats, high-fat salad dressing, and so on.

#2: The Keto Cleanse

The Keto Cleanse is the process of fully transitioning your body to burning fats for energy instead of deriving energy from carbohydrates by limiting the number of carbs you consume and increasing your fat intake. It trains your body and metabolism to behave in a new way, removes harmful toxins from the body, improves your physiological processes, and improves your mental focus. In addition, it trains your body to adapt to a new and healthy way of cooking and eating.

The keto cleanse lasts for 28 days for a very important reason. According to different scientific studies, if something is done every day for 28 days (or 4 weeks), it becomes a permanent habit. Therefore, a 28-day keto cleanse is a great jumpstart for the diet. It engraves the habit in your mind and helps you stick to the diet even after the 28 days are over.

This book also provides you with a meal plan that you can use as a guide. By following the meal plan closely, you take the guesswork and decision anxiety out of it. By the end of the 28 days, you will feel much more confident in making the diet your own and modifying it to suit your needs going forward.

#3: Keto Cooking

Many people think a keto diet is going to be restrictive. Well, I am here to tell you that the keto diet is among the least restrictive diets. That said, there are some keto cooking rules and guidelines that you need to follow to maximize your success in this diet. Most of what you eat, starts in your kitchen and you may be doing more harm than good if you're not following proper keto cooking guidelines.

Calculate: First and foremost, you need to start learning how to calculate the nutritional value of everything you consume. Keeping track of the calories and carbs going into your body is very important if you want to have an effective keto cleanse. Don't deceive yourself that you can measure the amount of food you eat by eyeballing it. That 6 ounces of bacon might end up being 10 ounces. The only way to be sure is by measuring it. You need to be strict with yourself and at first calculate the nutritional value of everything you ingest. Weigh and measure when you cook. Follow recipes precisely if you're relying on their nutritional content. It's all too easy to simply estimate or assume the nutritional value of what you're eating, but it's much better to be precise so you know how to budget your carbs and calories throughout the day.

Substitute: Next, you should find out some great carbohydrate alternatives. Instead of eating rice, try cauliflower rice. Instead of pasta, try vegetable noodles. Alternatively, you can try shiritaki noodles (tofu noodles), which are very keto friendly. Instead of cow's milk, you should try using alternatives like soy milk and almond milk. If you have a sweet tooth, find keto-friendly alternatives to indulge. At the same time, you should avoid things like grains, sugars, and processed foods. There are almost always keto-friendly substitutes available if you're creative enough.

Be Realistic: To increase your chances of success, you should also be realistic with yourself. Don't overestimate your commitment. If cooking every night is a problem for you, focus on meals that you can prepare ahead of time. If you think making new dishes every day is a challenge, you can master 10 or so dishes and repeat them if you don't mind less variety in your diet. You can keep your breakfasts simple and use a few recipes for breakfast every week.

#4 The Keto Kitchen

Once you start your keto cleanse, you will find yourself preparing your meals at home most of the time. To make this easier and more convenient for you, you need to invest in some kitchen tools and appliances. Below are some of the very basic tools and appliances that you need to make your keto experiments easier and more fun:

Food Scale

While it's possible to just have a "lazy keto" diet, where you just count your carbs and ignore the other details, your keto cleanse will be more effective when you are able to accurately track all your food intake. A food scale is the best way to keep track of everything you consume, instead of relying on estimates. Apart from tracking your food intake, a food scale is also an important cooking tool because you will need it to measure out various ingredients for your keto recipes.

Measuring Cups And Spoons

Apart from the measuring scale, a good keto kitchen should have quality measuring cups and spoons. These are good for measuring volumes of liquid ingredients as well as some dry ingredients like flours and sweeteners. When it comes to measuring cups and spoons, you can go with either plastic or stainless steel. Plastic is cheap, but stainless steel is more durable and less likely to stain.

Food Processor/Blender

Many keto recipes will also require a significant amount of food processing or blending. Instead of buying each appliance individually, it is better to buy an "all-in-one" food processor, blender, and drink mixer. This is more convenient and helps you save space in your kitchen.

Cast Iron Skillet

This is a tool you are going to use for a lot of your keto cooking. Cast iron skillets retain heat superbly, are non-stick, and can even be safely used in the oven. They last a long time and are well worth the investment.

Spiralizer

When you embark on your keto cleanse, you will quickly realize that spiralized veggies are a great, low-carb alternative to pasta. This makes it important for you to have a spiralizer in your kitchen. You can go with a cheap handheld spiralizer or opt for a more convenient but more expensive countertop version.

Silicone Baking Mats/Cups

While you will still require paper cup liners and parchment paper, the silicone versions are better because they are non-stick and can be safely used in the freezer/oven.

The above are not the only tools and appliances that you need in your keto kitchen, but they are some of the most basic that you should have before you embark on your keto cleanse.

#5: Keto Shopping

One of the advantages of undergoing keto cleansing is that you focus on eating real food instead of processed junk. The flip side is that you now have to do your own shopping for fresh foods, which might be a bit pricey. However, the following tips can keep your grocery budget in control:

1. **Keep it simple**. You don't have to experiment with fancy recipes every day. Instead, you should rely on recipes that require simple ingredients like vegetables, meats, and fats like olive oil or butter.
2. If possible, always **buy in bulk**. Warehouse retailers will give you bargains that are worth the membership charge. Why pay $8 for a pound of meat when you can get five pounds at $16 at the local warehouse store? All you need to do is to buy some decent reusable freezer containers and you can preserve your bulk purchases for longer.
3. Learn the **shelf life** of ingredients and plan your shopping accordingly. For instance, fresh herbs, fresh produce, and fresh meats have a short shelf life, so you should buy them with plans to use them soon, otherwise they will go bad in your fridge. Others like dairy products and eggs and non-perishables have a longer shelf life and can be bought in bulk and preserved for a long time.
4. Buy **fattier meat** cuts, as they are usually cheaper. This has an added advantage in keto cooking, since it allows you to increase your fat intake while managing your protein intake.
5. **Shop sales**. Nowadays, most supermarkets have sales circulars. Buying your groceries during sales can save you a good amount of money. Since you have access to the sale circular, the secret is to plan your meals around the sales.
6. **Buy in season**: Plan your meals around produce that is in season as it is going to be cheaper.

The above tips will help you save a significant amount of money on your keto shopping. It's important to have specific meals in mind when you're shopping for perishables and produce. That said, you should keep keto ingredients on hand to avoid slipping back to your high-carb ways. Some of the ingredients you should always have in your kitchen include:

Meats: Examples: Ground beef, chicken, duck, sausage, rib eye steak, pork, lamb chops, bacon, and various kinds of sea food.

Fruits and vegetables: Broccoli, cauliflower, cabbage, bell peppers, avocados, zucchini, onions, garlic, lettuce, cucumbers, berries, etc.

Dairy: Heavy cream, cream cheese, butter, hard cheeses, sour cream, eggs, etc.

Fats and oils: Olive oil, avocado oil, sesame oil, coconut oil, etc.

Miscellaneous: Mustard, vinegars, sugar-free salad dressing, olives, almond butter, ketogenic flours, sugar-free sauces, etc.

#6: Keto Meal Planning

The most challenging part for someone embarking on a keto cleanse is figuring out what to eat. Knowing what to eat each day can help you make a successful transition to the keto diet. On the other hand, starting a keto cleanse without a well laid-out plan is a good way of setting yourself up for failure. You need to follow a ketogenic meal plan to ensure that you do not backtrack. To make the transition easier for you, I have created a *28-day meal plan* that you can follow until keto becomes a habit for you. The meal plan gives you a variety of recipes to choose from, including **14 breakfasts, 28 lunches, and 28 dinners**.

With this meal plan, you will need to buy groceries at least once a week. To ensure you know what to buy each week, it's good to plan your menu a week earlier so that you do not find yourself without some of the ingredients that you might need.

This meal plan is not something you have to follow forever. You can add, subtract, and modify the recipes on this meal plan as you like. As you get deeper into your keto cleanse, eventually it will become second nature. You will instinctively know what to buy and how to plan your meals. However, it is always good to start with a guide to help you master the keto diet before you can own it and make it your own.

Part II: Recipes

Chapter 3: Meal Plan Overview

A meal plan is a guide of the meals you should cook for the duration of your keto cleanse. It is a calendar containing three meals (breakfast, lunch, and dinner) that you should eat each day. This meal plan contains 14 breakfasts you can then repeat for the second half of your 28-day keto cleanse. By following this meal plan, you will be able to stick to the keto diet by eliminating any guesswork and decision anxiety about what food you are supposed to eat. After the 28 days, the diet will become more instinctive and you can follow it through with your own keto-friendly recipes.

NOTE: this table follows the progression of the book in order that the recipes are listed:

    1). Breakfast: 14 recipes

    2). Lunch: 28 Recipes

    3). Dinner: 28 Recipes

Why only 14 recipes for breakfast? Breakfast is probably the meal you have the least time and energy for so we tried to keep it simple and limit it to 14 choices, for the remaining 14 days of the cleanse you can repeat any or all of the first 14 breakfast recipes.

ALSO: this table is a guide if you want to follow this meal plan to a T. Obviously depending on your schedule and your desire for simplicity vs. variety, you may decide to just stick to 10 or 15 recipes lunch and dinner recipes each and just repeat them. If you're up for the challenge, try to make all the recipes listed here for each of the days of your 28 day cleanse. If you desire simplicity, pick your favorite ones and just cycle them throughout the cleanse. Either way, you will have plenty of delicious options.

	Day 1	**Day 2**	**Day 3**	**Day 4**
Breakfast	Smoked Ham, Spinach, and Cheese Frittata Cups NC: 1.8	Almond and Sesame Bread NC: 2.7	Swiss Chard and Egg Pie NC: 4	Cream Cheese and Cinnamon Pancakes NC: 3
Lunch	Homemade Pork Tenderloin with Herbs NC: 0	Pasta with Mushrooms and Carrots NC: 4	Riced Cauliflower with Spicy Chicken NC: 13	Tuna and Avocado Salad NC: 11.5
Dinner	Keto Pork Lettuce Wraps NC: 2.5	Chorizo Stuffed Spaghetti Squash NC: 16.4	Sweet and Spicy Pork Roast NC: 1	Keto Beef Short Ribs NC: 6.1

	Day 5	**Day 6**	**Day 7**	**Day 8**
Breakfast	Vanilla and Coconut Waffle NC: 1.1	Bacon, Egg, and Mushroom Delight NC: 1.4	Cream Cheese and Pumpkin Muffins NC: 2.6	Keto Donuts NC: 1

Lunch	Fried Atlantic Cod Fillet *NC: 1*	Broccoli Salad with Bacon *NC: 10*	Bacon-Wrapped Chicken Breast *NC: 7*	Pork and Cabbage Casserole *NC: 8*
Dinner	Breaded Cod Fillet *NC: 5.7*	Haddock Fillet Cakes with Mayo Sauce *NC: 3.1*	Salmon Keto Poke *NC: 8.5*	Keto Steak Salad *NC: 8.3*

	Day 9	**Day 10**	**Day 11**	**Day 12**
Breakfast	Poppy and Flax Seed Muffins *NC: 2*	Keto Focaccia Bread *NC: 3*	Chia Seeds and Berries Smoothie *NC: 9*	Vanilla and Cream Crepe Cake *NC: 6*
Lunch	Thai Salad and Steak *NC: 4.6*	Spicy Marinara Meatballs *NC: 9*	Beef, Chicken, and Pistachio Terrine *NC: 2.6*	Spaghetti Squash Casserole *NC: 13*
Dinner	Baked Sea Bass *NC: 1.5*	Eggplant Parmesan *NC: 7.3*	Spicy Beef Stroganoff Stew *NC: 8.4*	Keto Beef Burgundy *NC: 6.9*

	Day 13	**Day 14**	**Day 15**	**Day 16**
Breakfast	Nutty Chocolate Breakfast Brownies *NC: 7.6*	Avocado and Spinach Smoothie *NC: 6*		
Lunch	Herb Dumplings with Braised Beef Stew *NC: 8*	Pork, Cheese, and Spinach Wraps *NC: 3*	Creamy Tuscan Chicken Cutlets *NC: 2.6*	Pork Chops with Mushroom Sauce *NC: 4*
Dinner	Beef Steak with Mustard Sauce *NC: 3.3*	Rutabaga Gratin *NC: 10.2*	Hot 'N' Creamy Chicken Paprika *NC: 4.4*	Keto Quiche Lorraine *NC: 8.8*

	Day 17	**Day 18**	**Day 19**	**Day 20**

Breakfast				
Lunch	Stir-Fried Beef and Peppers NC: 4.2	Creamy Asparagus Soup NC: 4.8	Keto Kale and Pork Chops NC: 2.2	Cheesy Spinach Stuffed Mushroom Caps NC: 2.2
Dinner	Keto Oxtail Stew NC: 8.2	Autumn Harvest Stew NC: 9.1	Chorizo Stuffed Zucchini NC: 7	Egg and Bacon Stuffed Zucchini NC: 8

	Day 21	**Day 22**	**Day 23**	**Day 24**
Breakfast				
Lunch	Goat Cheese Burgers NC: 7.3	Mediterranean Chicken and Veggie Delight NC: 6.9	Focaccia Kale Salad NC: 4.76	Spinach, Bacon, and Mushroom Frittata NC: 4.76
Dinner	Keto Spinach Omelet NC: 7	Watercress Bisque NC: 6.8	Eggplant Lasagna NC: 8.7	Chorizo Tex Mex Stew NC: 6.4

	Day 25	**Day 26**	**Day 27**	**Day 28**
Breakfast				
Lunch	Lemon-Stuffed Grilled Trout NC: 2.1	Creamy Cauliflower Masala NC: 9.9	Brined Chicken Drumsticks NC: 2	Extra Krispy Chicken Wings with Sauce NC: 3.1
Dinner	Red Gazpacho with Cream NC: 8.5	Cauliflower Avgolemono Soup NC: 6	Thai Fried Noodles and Prawns NC: 8.4	Creamy Spinach and Salmon NC: 3.7

Chapter 4: Breakfast Recipes

Thought you had to say goodbye to waffles, pancakes, coffee cake, bread (especially breakfast breads) when you started the keto diet? Many of the following recipes will show you just how wrong you were — you will feel like you're cheating on your diet. The amazing thing about many of the following recipes is that you can make them ahead and just store them for a quick grab and go as you run out the door in the morning. What could be easier than that?

Smoked Ham, Spinach, And Cheese Frittata Cups

Yield: 12 cups
Ingredients:
7 oz smoked ham, chopped
6 large eggs
1 cup spinach leaves, finely chopped
½ cup Mexican shredded cheese
¼ tsp Himalayan sea salt
2 cloves garlic, minced
1 tsp black pepper powder
¼ tsp ground chili powder
1 tsp fresh rosemary, chopped

Method:

1. Preheat your oven to 350 degrees Fahrenheit. Use parchment paper to line a large muffin pan that holds 12 cups.
2. In a large bowl, mix the chopped spinach leaves, ham, cheese, rosemary, and garlic together. Stir well to ensure even distribution.
3. Take another mixing bowl and pour in the eggs, sea salt, chili powder, and black pepper. Whisk well until you get a frothy mixture. Pour the mixture into the bowl containing ham and spinach mixture. Mix well.
4. Pour this mixture into the 12 muffin cups. Don't fill to the top. Only fill ¾ of each cup.
5. Place the muffin pan into the oven and cook for 25 minutes. The top of the muffins should be slightly colored.
6. Let the muffins cool for five minutes and then remove the frittatas from the cups.
7. Serve either hot or cold sprinkled with shredded coconut.

Nutritional Values Per Serving:
- Calories – 64
- Fat – 4 g
- Protein – 5.6 g

16

- Carbs – 1.8 g

Almond And Sesame Bread

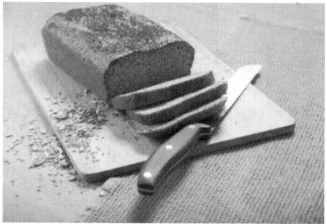

Yield: 1 loaf of 12 slices
Ingredients:
2 cups water
2 large eggs
6 large egg whites
5.3 oz almond flour
4.2 oz sesame seed flour
2.1 oz coconut flour
1.4 oz. psyllium husk powder
1 tbsp gluten-free baking powder
½ tsp sea salt
Method:
1. Preheat the oven to 350 degrees F.
2. Take a mixing bowl and combine the egg whites and whole eggs. Use a fork to mix the ingredients and then set the bowl aside. (The reason egg whites are used instead of all whole eggs is because the bread will not rise if there are too many yolks in it).
3. Pour all the different flours, powders, and sea salt into a large bowl and mix well. Ensure that there is even mixing. Pour the egg mixture into the dry ingredients and use a mixer to create thick dough. Bring the water to a boil, pour it into the dough and continue mixing. Make sure there is an even consistency.
4. Line a loaf tin using parchment paper. Grease the tin lightly with ghee to make sure that the parchment paper sticks well to the tin. When cutting the parchment paper, cut two strips that are long and large enough to hang over the sides of the loaf tin. This will help you when removing the bread from the tin.
5. Put the dough in the lined loaf tin and place it in the oven. Bake the bread for a maximum of 90 minutes.

6. When ready, remove the tin from the oven and use the parchment paper to take out the bread. Allow the bread to sit on a cooling rack to prevent the sides from becoming moist.
7. When the bread has cooled, cut it into 12 slices.
8. Top a slice with butter, cheese, and ham to make a sandwich.
9. Serve and enjoy!

Tip: Place any leftover slices in freezer bags and put in the freezer for up to three months. Whenever you want to eat them, defrost the slices or warm them up in the toaster, hot pan, or oven.

Nutritional Values Per Serving:
- Calories – 135
- Fat – 9.1 g
- Protein – 8.8 g
- Net carbs – 2.7 g
- Fiber – 5.4 g

Swiss Chard And Egg Pie

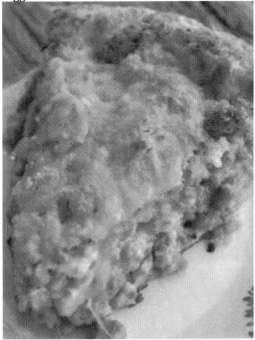

Yield: 8 servings/wedges
Ingredients:
8 cups Swiss chard, chopped
1 lb sausage
3 eggs
½ cup chopped onions
2 cups ricotta cheese

18

¼ cup parmesan, shredded
1 cup mozzarella, shredded
1 tbsp olive oil
⅛ tsp ground nutmeg
1 clove garlic
Salt and pepper, to taste

Method:
1. Preheat the oven to 350 degrees F.
2. Place a large pan over medium-low heat and pour the olive oil into it. Sauté the onions and garlic until soft.
3. Pour in the Swiss chard and cook until the stems turn soft and leaves become wilted. Remove the pan from heat and let it cool.
4. As the chard cools, take a large mixing bowl and pour in the eggs, ricotta, mozzarella, and parmesan. Mix thoroughly before stirring in the sautéed Swiss chard.
5. Take your pie tin and squeeze the sausage into it uniformly. Pour the filling into the pie tin and place the container on a cookie sheet. Bake in the oven until firm.
6. Serve with extra cheese on top if desired.

Nutritional Values Per Serving
- Calories – 344
- Fat – 27 g
- Protein – 23 g
- Net carbs – 4 g

Cream Cheese And Cinnamon Pancakes

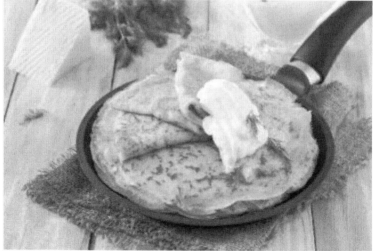

Yield: 4 servings
Ingredients:
2 large eggs
2 oz cream cheese

½ tsp cinnamon

1 tsp sugar substitute

Method:

1. Place all the ingredients into a blender and mix them until you achieve a smooth consistency.
2. Let the mixture sit for two minutes to allow bubbles to settle.
3. Place a non-stick pan over medium heat and use some butter to grease the surface. Pour ¼ of the mixture into the pan.
4. Cook one side until golden and then flip over. Cook the other side for one minute.
5. Repeat the process using the remaining batter.
6. Serve with sour cream and fresh dill.

Nutritional Values Per Serving

- Calories – 344
- Fat – 29 g
- Protein – 17 g
- Net carbs – 3 g

Vanilla And Coconut Waffles

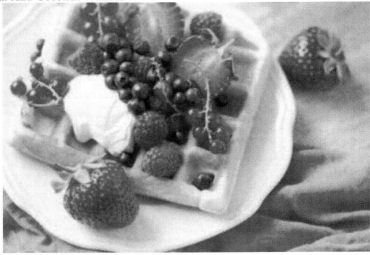

Yield: 8 servings

Ingredients:

7 tbsp coconut flour

5 tbsp full-fat cream

2 tsp baking powder

3 tsp vanilla

8 eggs

2 sticks of butter, melted

Method:

1. Separate the egg whites and the egg yolks into two bowls.
2. Fluff up the egg whites in the first bowl using a whisk.
3. Pour the butter into the second bowl with the egg yolks. Then add the vanilla and full-fat cream. Mix thoroughly.

4. Gently pour the egg whites into the second bowl. Ensure that you maintain the fluffiness of the egg whites.
5. Warm up the waffle maker and then pour in enough batter for one waffle.
6. Cook until the waffle turns golden.
7. Repeat using the remaining batter.
8. Serve with berries and sour cream or unsweetened whipped topping if desired.

Nutritional Values Per Serving:
- Calories – 280
- Fat – 26 g
- Protein – 7 g
- Fiber – 2 g
- Net carbs – 1.1 g

Bacon, Egg, And Mushroom Delight

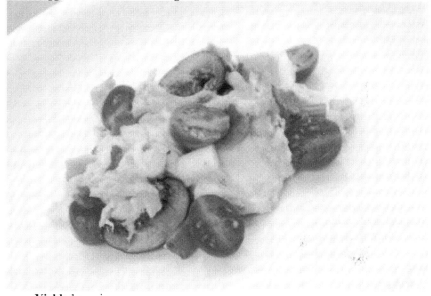

Yield: 1 serving
Ingredients:
2 slices turkey bacon
3 Bella mushrooms
½ cup cheddar cheese, shredded
2 large eggs
¼ cup green peppers
1 ½ tbsp extra virgin olive oil
3 grape tomatoes, halved

Method:
1. Chop the bacon, mushrooms, and green peppers and set aside.

2. Pour half a tablespoon of the extra virgin olive oil into a frying pan and sauté the chopped bacon, mushrooms, and green peppers.
3. Take a mixing bowl, crack the eggs into it, and whisk thoroughly.
4. Place a second pan over medium heat and pour one tablespoon of olive oil. Then scramble the eggs. Add some salt and pepper, to taste.
5. Pour the sautéed bacon and vegetable mix over the cooking eggs, and then top off with the cheddar cheese. Mix well.
6. Serve hot with the halved grape tomatoes.

Nutritional Values Per Serving:

- Calories – 570
- Fat – 53 g
- Protein – 41 g
- Net carbs – 1.4 g

Pumpkin Cream Cheese Muffins

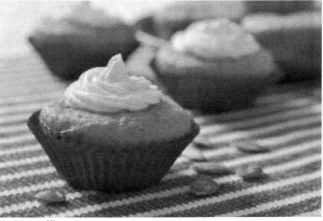

Yield: 20 muffins
Ingredients:
For Muffins:
1 cup pumpkin puree
6 eggs
2 tbsp sour cream
2 tbsp butter
1 tbsp pumpkin pie spice
¾ cup coconut flour
½ cup coconut oil
1 ½ tsp baking powder
1 ½ tsp vanilla
½ tsp salt
For Filling:
½ tsp vanilla
1 tbsp heavy whipped cream
3 oz cream cheese
Method:

22

1. Preheat oven to 350 degrees F.
2. Place a pan over medium-low heat and melt the butter and coconut oil.
3. Crack the eggs in a mixing bowl and add the pumpkin puree, vanilla, sour cream and pumpkin spice. Whisk the mixture well.
4. Pour the melted butter and coconut oil over the mixture.
5. Take a separate mixing bowl and mix the coconut flour, baking powder, and salt.
6. Pour the flour mixture into the first mixing bowl. Mix thoroughly.
7. Make the filling by pouring its ingredients into a blender. Mix well.
8. Grease muffin tins, line them with parchment paper, and then fill them with the batter.
9. Use a spoon to scoop the filling over the top of the batter of each muffin tin. Leave about half of the filling for later.
10. Use a toothpick to swirl the filling into the batter.
11. Place in the oven for 25 minutes.
12. Remove from the oven and top off with the remaining cream filling.
13. Serve.

Nutritional Values Per Serving:
- Calories – 147
- Fat – 13 g
- Protein – 3.5 g
- Net carbs – 2.6 g

Keto Donuts

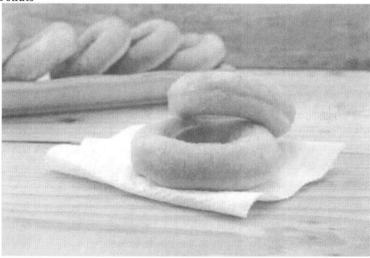

Yield: 4 servings
Ingredients:
1 tsp vanilla extract
1 tsp coconut flour
4 tbsp almond flour
1 tsp baking flour

3 oz cream cheese
3 large eggs
Coconut oil for cooking

Method:
1. Take a large mixing bowl and pour all the ingredients into it.
2. Using an immersion blender, mix the ingredients thoroughly.
3. Use the coconut oil to grease the surface of the donut maker. Once you have heated up the donut-maker, pour the batter into every well.
4. Cook the first side for three minutes before flipping over. Then cook the other side for two minutes.
5. Remove the donuts and repeat the process with the leftover batter.
6. Serve. You can dust w/powdered artificial sweetener of choice, or mix cinnamon and granulated stevia and roll donuts in cinnamon "sugar" mixture (make sure to calculate amounts and update nutrition values accordingly)

Nutritional Values Per Serving:
- Calories – 32
- Fats – 2.8 g
- Protein – 1.5 g
- Net carbs – 0.3 g

Poppy And Flax Seed Muffins

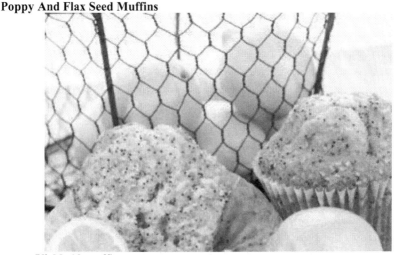

Yield: 12 muffins
Ingredients:
3 eggs
¼ cup flaxseed meal
2 tbsp poppy seeds
¾ cup almond flour
1 tsp baking powder
¼ cup heavy cream

¼ butter, melted
1 tsp vanilla extract
2 tbsp lemon juice
Zest of 1 lemon
20 drops liquid Stevia

Method:

1. Preheat oven to 350 degrees F.
2. Take a mixing bowl and combine the flaxseed meal, poppy seeds, and almond flour. Mix them together using a fork.
3. Crack the eggs in a separate bowl and add the melted butter and heavy cream. Whisk the mixture well.
4. Pour the liquid mixture into the bowl containing the dry ingredients. Mix them well until you get a smooth consistency with no lumps whatsoever.
5. Then add the vanilla extract, liquid Stevia, lemon juice, lemon zest, and baking powder. Mix thoroughly.
6. Get 12 silicone cupcake molds and pour the batter into the molds. Try to keep the level of the batter equal in every mold. Alternatively, you can use a muffin pan.
7. Place the molds or pan in the oven and bake for about 20 minutes. The top of the muffins should be slightly brown.
8. Remove the muffins and allow them to cool for 10 minutes.
9. Serve! If you like, you can slice the muffins in half and stick a pad of butter in between the slices.

Nutritional Values Per Muffin:

- Calories – 100
- Fats – 11.7 g
- Protein – 4 g
- Net carbs – 1.7 g
- Fiber – 1.6 g

Keto Breakfast Focaccia Bread

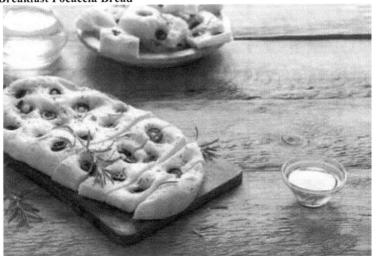

Yield: 6 servings
Ingredients:
1.8 oz coconut flour
1 tsp gluten-free baking powder
4 large eggs
2 ½ tbsp psyllium husks
1.8 oz plain whole milk yogurt
½ tsp salt
For Topping:
2 tbsp extra virgin olive oil
2 tbsp mixed herbs (sage, rosemary, thyme, etc)
¼ Kalamata olives, sliced
Salt, to taste
Method:
1. Preheat the oven to 375 degrees F.
2. Take a large mixing bowl and crack the eggs into it. Add the yogurt and whisk together.
3. Then add the coconut flour, psyllium husks, and baking powder. Stir until the mixture forms thick dough.
4. Use parchment paper to line a baking sheet. Place the ball of dough on the baking sheet and mould the dough into a rectangular shape about a half-inch thick.
5. Place a small pot over low heat and add the olive oil, herbs, and salt. Heat the herbs until they release a fragrance.
6. Sprinkle the dough with the olive oil and top with the herbs and olives.
7. Place the dough in the oven and bake for about 15 minutes.

8. Slice and serve. The bread can be stored at room temperature for a maximum of three days. (It's delicious toasted with a fried egg on top ☺)

Nutritional Values Per Serving:
- Calories – 144
- Fat – 10.9 g
- Protein – 6.6 g
- Net carbs – 1.8 g
- Fiber – 3 g

Chia Seeds And Berries Smoothie

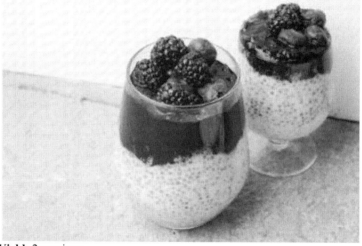

Yield: 2 servings
Ingredients:
½ cup blackberries,
½ cup blueberries
4 tbsp chia seeds
2 cups unsweetened coconut milk
Method:
1. Pour the coconut milk, chia seeds, and berries into a food processor.
2. Blend the mixture until all the berries have dissolved. The mixture will turn a purplish color.
3. Place in the fridge for an hour.
4. Serve with a topping of more berries. Enjoy!

Nutritional Values Per Serving:
- Calories – 762
- Fat – 61.4 g
- Protein – 16 g
- Net carbs – 10 g
- Fiber – 18 g

Vanilla Cream Crepe "Coffee Cake"

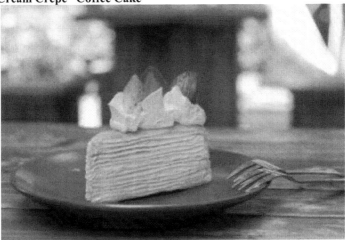

Yield: 4 servings
Ingredients:
For The Crepes:
2 large eggs
¼ cup almond flour
2 tbsp butter
2 oz cream cheese
1 tsp unsweetened soy milk
For The Topping And Filling;
 6 large strawberries
½ tsp vanilla extract
4 oz heavy cream
Method:
1. The first step is to make the batter for the crepes. Break the eggs into a food processor and then add the cream cheese and almond flour. Mix the ingredients well. Pour in the soy milk and process the ingredients until you get a smooth consistency. Add more soy milk if necessary to thin the mixture.
2. Place a frying pan over medium heat. Melt some of the butter in the pan and grease the surface evenly. When the butter becomes hot, pour two tablespoons of the batter into the pan and swirl it to ensure a thin layer.
3. When the edges of the crepe turn brown, use a spatula to flip it over to the other side. Cook until the crepe turns slightly brown and then remove it from the pan.
4. Use the remaining batter to make the rest of the crepes. There should be enough to make five more. Allow all the crepes to cool.
5. As the crepes cool, prepare the filling. Pour the heavy cream and vanilla extract into the food processor and mix well. If you prefer, you can add some artificial sweetener to sweeten the filling.
6. Arrange the crepes in a neat stack and then use a sharp knife to cut the stack in half.

7. Take one crepe (or rather half-crepe) and place it on a serving plate. Spread some of the cream and vanilla filling over the top of the crepe, making sure that it is a thin layer. Take another crepe, stack it on top of the first one, and spread another thin layer of filling. Repeat the process until you have used all the crepes.
8. When you are done, put the crepes in the fridge for about an hour.
9. Meanwhile, slice the strawberries into halves.
10. After one hour, remove the crepes and top off with some cream and the halved strawberries.

Nutritional Values Per Serving:
- Calories – 292
- Fat – 28 g
- Protein – 6 g
- Net carbs – 6 g
- Fiber – 1 g

Nutty Chocolate Breakfast Brownies

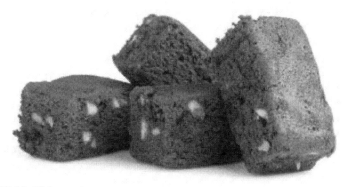

Yield: 20 brownies
Ingredients:
6 oz dark Belgian chocolate
3 tbsp hazelnuts, crushed
8 tbsp unsalted butter
4 large eggs
2 ½ c. almond flour
½ tsp. baking powder
½ tsp. vanilla extract
¾ cup erythritol
A pinch of salt
Method:
1. Preheat oven to 320 degrees F.
2. Chop the chocolate and butter into chunks and place in a bowl that is microwave-safe. Microwave the chocolate and butter for around 90 seconds. Remove the bowl and stir the mixture to ensure a smooth consistency. Then allow the mixture to cool.

3. Take a large mixing bowl and crack the eggs into it. Add the vanilla extract, erythritol, and salt, and mix for about three minutes using a whisk. (Salt tends to improve the flavor of chocolate brownies).
4. Pour the chocolate-butter mixture as you whisk gently.
5. Get another mixing bowl and pour in the almond flour and baking powder. Stir well.
6. Use a rubber spatula to pour the flour mixture into the chocolate mixture.
7. Line a large baking pan with parchment paper. Pour the mixture into the pan and use the spatula to spread it evenly.
8. Sprinkle the crushed hazelnuts all over the mixture.
9. Put the baking pan in the oven for around 30 minutes (If you want the brownies to come out fudgy, reduce the time to 25 minutes). It is important that you do not bake the brownies for too long. Use a toothpick to check the center of the brownies.
10. When ready, remove the baking pan from the oven. Lift the parchment paper and the whole batch off the pan and set aside to cool. Then slice into 20 brownies of equal size.
11. Serve and enjoy!

Nutritional Values Per Brownie:
- Calories – 110
- Fat – 9.2 g
- Protein – 3.3 g
- Net carbs – 7.6g
- Fiber – 3.7 g

Avocado and Spinach Smoothie

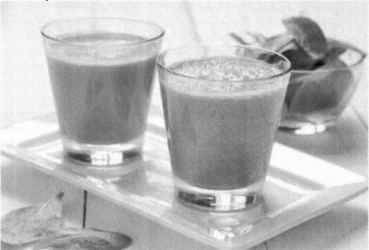

Yield: 1 serving
Ingredients:
0.5 oz fresh spinach
2.6 oz avocado
½ cup coconut milk

½ tsp vanilla powder
5 drops liquid Stevia
1 tbsp extra virgin coconut oil
½ cup water and some ice cubes

Method:

1. Slice the avocado in half and remove the seed.
2. Pour all the other ingredients into a blender.
3. Scoop the flesh of the avocado into the blender and mix everything together.
4. Toss in the ice and blend until smooth.
5. Pour in a glass and enjoy!

Nutritional Values Per Serving:

- Calories – 468
- Fat – 48.2
- Protein – 4.2
- Net carbs – 6 g
- Fiber – 5.4 g

Chapter Five: Lunch Recipes

There are many diverse recipes included here. Some are quick and easy, some are a little more labor intensive and fancy, and many are great to prep ahead for portioning out and taking to work with you. Remember, you certainly don't have to make all these recipes for your cleanse. If it's easier for you to find 10 or 15 recipes you really like, just repeat them for the remainder of the cleanse, these recipes are meant to give you many diverse options.

Homemade Pork Tenderloin With Herbs

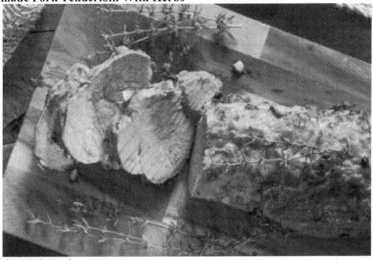

Yield: 2 servings
Ingredients:
1 tbsp olive oil
1 lb pork tenderloin
Thyme, parsley and rosemary for topping
Salt and black pepper, to taste
Method:
1. Heat a pan over medium heat and pour in the olive oil.
2. Using a sharp knife, cut the pork tenderloin into two halves.
3. When the oil becomes hot, place the tenderloin in the pan. As you cook the meat, make sure that you keep flipping them over so that each side cooks well.
4. Take a reading of the internal temperature of the tenderloin using a meat thermometer. The ideal reading should be just less than 145 degrees F (63 degrees C).
5. Remove the tenderloin from the pan and set the two halves aside. Allow them to cool.
6. Once they have cooled, cut the tenderloin into slices and sprinkle the herbs over the meat.
7. Serve and enjoy! (this is great to make ahead, and then take with you to work)
Nutritional Values Per Serving:
- Calories – 330
- Fat – 15 g
- Protein – 47 g
- Net carbs – 0 g

Pasta With Mushrooms And Carrots

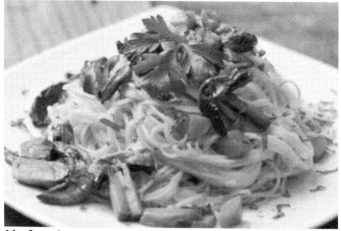

Yields: 2 servings
Ingredients:
3 cups mushrooms
2 cups carrots, diced
2 packs tofu noodles
2 cloves garlic
1 tsp almond flour
2 tbsp butter
¾ tub heavy cream
¼ tsp black pepper
¼ tsp sea alt
A pinch of dried parsley
Fresh parsley, chopped
Olive oil
Method:
1. Drain the tofu noodles and rinse. Set the pasta aside.
2. Place a frying pan over medium heat and melt the butter. Add the carrots and garlic and cook for about one minute.
3. Place the mushrooms in the frying pan. Use a spatula to swirl the mushrooms around to get an even coating of the oil. Cook for about five minutes and make sure to stir regularly. The mushrooms should turn a golden-brown color.
4. Scoop out the mushrooms and leave the oil in the pan.
5. Pour the almond flour, cream, and parsley into the pan and stir. Mix the ingredients with the oil in the pan.
6. Sprinkle some salt and pepper into the pan and continue heating for two more minutes.
7. Pour the pasta and mushrooms into the pan and mix well.
8. Serve hot topped with parsley.
Nutritional Values Per Serving:
- Calories – 237
- Fat – 20 g

- Protein – 6 g
- Net carbs – 4 g
- Fiber – 10 g

Riced Cauliflower With Spicy Chicken

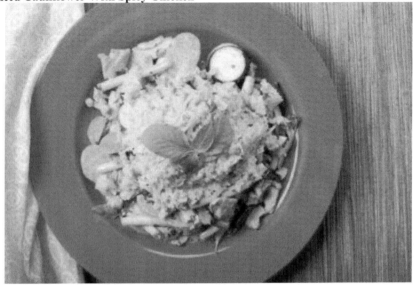

Yield: 4 servings
Ingredients:
4 chicken breasts, cooked and cubed
3 eggs
1 head cauliflower
1 tbsp coconut aminos
1 tbsp grated ginger
½ cup cilantro, chopped
3 chilis, chopped
3 cloves garlic, minced
Coconut oil for cooking
Salt, to taste
Method:
1. Take the cauliflower florets and put them in a blender. Process them until the texture of the cauliflower pieces resembles rice. If not all the florets will fit in the blender, process them in batches.
2. Take a large pan and place it over medium heat. Melt the coconut oil in the pan and then cook the riced cauliflower. You may have to cook in batches. Just make sure you stir regularly.
3. Heat another pan and melt some coconut oil. Scramble the eggs and then pour them over the cauliflower rice. Keep cooking the cauliflower.
4. Add the ginger, chilis, and garlic.
5. When the cauliflower has turned soft, add the chicken pieces.

6. Pour in the coconut aminos and sprinkle some salt. Mix well.
7. Use the chopped cilantro as garnish.
8. Serve.

Nutritional Values Per Serving:
- Calories – 350
- Fat – 11 g
- Protein – 55 g
- Net carbs – 13 g
- Fiber – 4 g

Tuna And Avocado Salad

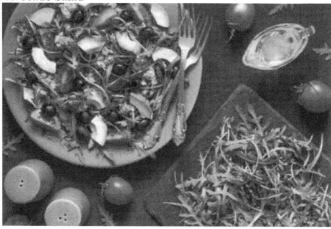

Yield: 1 serving
Ingredients:
6 oz tuna
Salad greens
½ large avocado, sliced
1 tbsp lemon juice
1 tbsp mayo
1 tbsp mustard
Sea salt and black pepper

Method:
1. Place the slices of avocado in a bowl and pour in the lemon juice.
2. Take another bowl and flake the tuna. Then add the mayo and mustard. Mix thoroughly.
3. Pour the tuna mixture over the avocado slices.
4. Prepare the salad greens and place in a large mixing bowl. Then pour the tuna and avocado into the bowl.
5. Add the salt and pepper to taste and toss.
6. Serve.

Nutritional Values Per Serving:
- Calories – 480
- Fat – 40 g

- Protein – 45 g
- Net carbs – 11.5 g
- Fiber – 8 g

Fried Atlantic Cod Fillet

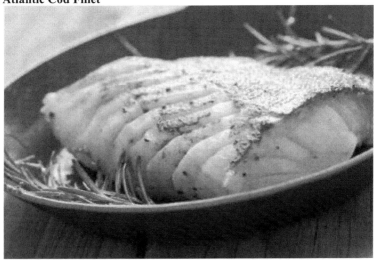

Yield: 4 servings
Ingredients:
4 cod fillets
3 tbsp ghee
6 garlic cloves, minced
Salt and pepper, to taste
Method:
1. Take a large pan and place it over medium heat.
2. Heat the ghee in the pan until it melts. Then add half of the minced garlic.
3. Place the fish fillets in the pan and sprinkle some salt over the fish.
4. As the fish cooks on one side, the fillet should become solid white halfway through the side. When you see this, flip the fillet over and add the leftover garlic.
5. Fry the cod fillets until the whole fish becomes flaky and solid white.
6. Serve with the garlic and ghee remaining in the pan. You can also use some rosemary as topping.
Nutritional Values Per Serving:
- Calories – 160
- Fat – 7 g
- Proteins – 21 g
- Net carbs – 1 g

Broccoli Salad With Bacon

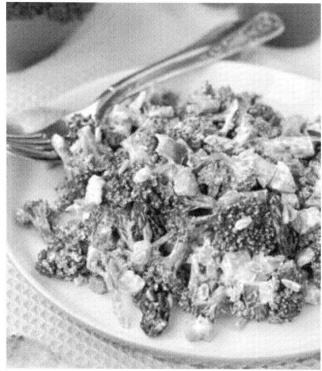

Yield: 6 servings
Ingredients:
1 lb broccoli florets
20 slices of bacon, chopped
2 onions, diced
1 cup coconut cream
Salt and pepper, to taste
Sunflower seeds for topping
Method:
1. Place a pan over medium heat and fry the pieces of bacon.
2. Remove the bacon and use the fat left in the pan to sauté the onions.
3. Boil the broccoli florets until they turn soft.
4. In a large mixing bowl, pour in the broccoli, onions, and bacon. Then pour the coconut cream over the bacon salad.
5. Sprinkle some salt to add flavor and top off with some sunflower seeds.
6. Serve and enjoy!
Nutritional Values Per Serving:
- Calories – 280
- Fat – 26 g
- Protein – 7 g

- Carbs – 10 g
- Fiber – 3 g

Bacon-Wrapped Chicken Breast

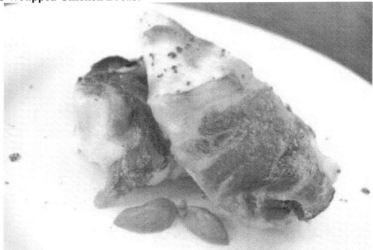

Yield: 2 servings
Ingredients:
2 chicken breasts
4 slices of bacon
3 tbsp garlic powder
Method:
1. Preheat oven to 400 degrees F.
2. Pour garlic powder into a bowl and dip the chicken breasts into the powder. Make sure each piece is evenly coated by the garlic powder.
3. Use 2 slices of bacon to wrap each of the chicken breasts.
4. Take a baking tray and line its surface with aluminum foil. Then place the chicken breasts on the tray, separated by a bit of space.
5. Place the baking tray in the oven and let the chicken cook for about 15 minutes. Then turn the breasts over. When the bacon becomes crispy, remove the tray from the oven.
6. Serve and enjoy! (These are also great to make in batches and portion out for lunches)
Nutritional Values Per Serving:
- Calories – 443
- Fat – 21 g
- Protein – 51 g
- Net carbs – 7 g
- Fiber – 1 g

Pork And Cabbage Casserole

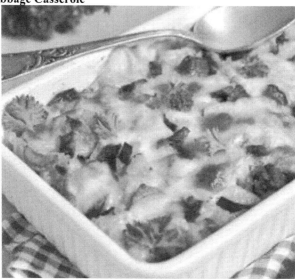

Yield: 8 servings
Ingredients:
14 oz smoked pork chops, cubed
Medium-sized green cabbage, cored and sliced
1 cup onion
1 ½ cups crushed tomatoes
14 ½ oz can diced tomatoes
¼ cup parsley, chopped
1 ½ cups Mozzarella cheese
4 cloves garlic, minced
1 red bell pepper
2 tbsp organic butter
2 tbsp olive oil
Black pepper and sea salt, to taste
Method:
1. Preheat oven to 400 degrees F.
2. Place a large skillet on medium heat and heat the butter and olive oil
3. When the butter has melted, toss in the cabbage slices, bell pepper, garlic, onion, black pepper, and salt. Sauté the ingredients until the cabbage wilts and the other veggies become tender. This should take about 10 minutes.
4. Add the crushed tomatoes, diced tomatoes, and smoked pork chop cubes. Sauté for another 10 minutes.
5. Pour the mixture into a casserole dish and grate the cheese over the dish.
6. Place the casserole dish into the oven and bake for about 15 minutes.
7. Remove the casserole and sprinkle the chopped parsley over it.
8. Serve and enjoy! (This one is great because you make a big batch and then you have lunch every day for that whole week)

Nutritional Values Per Serving:
- Calories – 333
- Fat – 25 g
- Protein – 15.5 g
- Net carbs – 8 g
- Fiber – 3.75 g

Thai Steak Salad

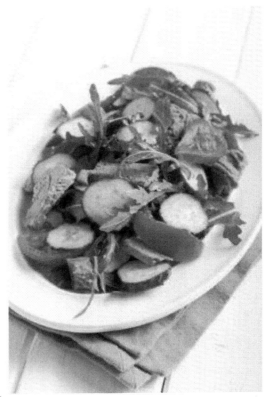

Yield: 2 servings
Ingredients:
2.5 oz salad greens
4 grape tomatoes, halved
4 radishes, sliced
2 cucumbers, sliced
½ lb beef steak
½ tbsp olive oil
½ tbsp lemon juice
½ red bell pepper, sliced
¼ cup soy sauce (gluten free)
Salt, to taste
Avocado oil for cooking

Method:
1. Marinate the steak using the soy sauce.
2. Take a large mixing bowl and put the salad greens, cucumbers, tomatoes, radishes, and bell peppers in it. Toss the salad with the olive oil, lemon juice, and salt.
3. Heat the avocado oil in a pan and fry the steak according to your preference. Then set the steak aside to cool for about one minute.
4. Meanwhile, place the salad on two serving plates.
5. Use a sharp knife to cut the steak into slices and share out among the two salads, then serve.

Nutritional Values Per Serving:
- Calories – 532
- Fat – 37.1 g
- Protein – 33.3 g
- Net carbs – 4.6 g
- Fiber – 2.3 g

Spicy Marinara Meatballs

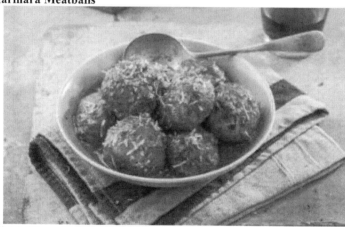

Yield: 25 meatballs/4 servings
Ingredients:
For The Meatballs:
1 large egg
1.1 lb ground beef
1 cup mozzarella, diced (low moisture)
½ cup almond flour
1 tsp dried thyme
1 tsp dried oregano
2 cloves garlic, minced
Freshly ground black pepper
Sea salt, to taste
Fresh basil for garnish
For The Marinara Sauce:

1 cup tomatoes
¼ cup extra virgin olive oil
¼ cup tomato paste, unsweetened
1 cup fresh basil
1 small white onion
2 cloves garlic
Freshly ground black pepper
¼ tsp sea salt

Method:

1. Preheat the oven to 450 degrees F.
2. Slice the mozzarella into 25 pieces of equal size. Put the cheese in the freezer for about 45 minutes. This is so it won't leak out while baking the meatballs.
3. Meanwhile, take a large mixing bowl and combine the ground beef, oregano, minced garlic, almond flour, thyme, black pepper, and salt. Crack the egg into the bowl and mix everything well using your hands.
4. Make 25 balls of meat from the beef mixture. Then take the pieces of cheese out of the freezer.
5. Use your hands to flatten every ball of meat. Take a piece of cheese and place it in the center of a flattened meatball. Then fold the meat over the piece of cheese. Repeat this for every meatball.
6. Roll each meatball with your hands to ensure that the meat totally covers the cheese.
7. Take a baking tray and line it with some parchment paper. Place the meatballs on the parchment paper and put the baking tray in the oven. The meatballs should bake for 15 minutes.
8. As the meatballs are cooking, prepare your marinara sauce.
9. To make the sauce, first wash and drain the basil and tomatoes. Then peel the garlic and onion.
10. Put all the ingredients for the sauce into a food processor. Blend the ingredients until you get a smooth consistency.
11. If you don't want chunks of onion or garlic in the sauce, you can mash the garlic and dice the onion before processing the ingredients. Alternatively, if you prefer your sauce to have a chunky texture, set aside some tomatoes and basil, dice them, and toss them into the smooth sauce after processing.
12. Take a large saucepan, place it over medium heat, and heat the marinara sauce.
13. The meatballs should be ready by now. Remove the baking tray from the oven and dip the meatballs into the saucepan.
14. Use a spatula to stir the meatballs around the sauce. Make sure that every meatball is covered in the marinara sauce.
15. Chop the fresh basil and garnish the meatballs.
16. Serve and enjoy!

Tip: You can also keep the marinara sauce in a separate bowl and simply dip the meatballs into the sauce. To preserve marinara sauce, pour it into an airtight container and place it in the refrigerator. It will last up to a week.

Nutritional Values Per Meatball:

- Calories – 117

- Fat – 9.3 g
- Protein – 7 g
- Net carbs – 9 g
- Fiber – 0.5 g

Beef, Chicken, and Pistachio Terrine

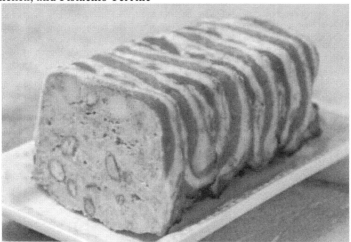

Yield: 6 servings
Ingredients:
17 oz chicken thighs, skin removed
4.2 oz beef, minced
2 cloves garlic, minced
1 leek, finely sliced
1 large egg
12 slices Prosciutto di Parma
2 tsp fresh thyme
2 tbsp ghee
1 tbsp sage, chopped
3 mushrooms, thinly sliced
4 oz raw pistachio nuts, shelled and roughly chopped
¼ tsp black pepper
½ tsp pink Himalayan salt
Method:
1. Preheat oven to 355 degrees F.
2. Put half of the chicken into a food processor. Blend the chicken to create a mince. Chop the other half of the chicken thighs into half-inch cubes.
3. Take a large mixing bowl and place both the minced and cubed chicken. Add the minced beef and mix all the meat together well.
4. Take a small pan and place over medium heat. Melt the ghee and cook the garlic, leeks, sage, and thyme. When the leek mixture becomes soft, pour it in a bowl and set aside to cool.

5. Using the same frying pan, sauté the mushrooms until they turn a nice brown color. If necessary, add a bit of ghee to fry the mushrooms well. Then set the mushrooms aside in a separate bowl and let them cool.

6. Crack the egg into the large bowl containing the chicken and beef mixture. Then add the leek mixture and pistachio nuts. Mix well and season with black pepper and salt.

7. Get a loaf tin and line it with foil, making sure that a lot of foil hangs over the sides. Place the prosciutto slices at the bottom and along the sides of the loaf tin. Make sure that the slices hang over the edges of the tin.

8. Use a spoon to scoop half of the chicken and beef mixture into the loaf tin. Press the mixture down hard to keep it compact.

9. Spread the mushrooms all over the top of the mixture and then add the remaining half of the chicken and beef mixture. Press the mixture down to keep it compact.

10. Gently fold the prosciutto slices over the top of the mixture. Then fold the foil to cover the prosciutto.

11. Place the loaf tin in the oven for about an hour. When the terrine is cooked, remove the loaf tin from the oven and put it in the sink.

12. Press down on the terrine using another loaf tin to get rid of any juices. You can also place tomato cans in the loaf tin to add extra weight. Whatever method you use, just make sure that all the juices are released from the terrine.

13. With the added weight still on top, place the tin containing the terrine on a shallow tray. Then put everything in the fridge overnight.

14. When you are ready, remove the tin from the fridge and then take the terrine out of the loaf tin. Gently remove the foil. You will see a gel-like liquid around the terrine. Wipe this off using a damp paper towel.

15. Use a sharp knife to cut the terrine into slices.

16. Serve cold with low-carb veggies (cucumber, radishes, peppers, tomatoes, and red onions) or drizzle some extra virgin olive oil and serve with dressed greens. The terrine can last up to four days in the refrigerator.

Nutritional Values Per Serving:
- Calories - 243
- Fat – 12 g
- Protein – 29.2 g
- Net carbs – 2.6 g
- Fiber – 0.6 g

Spaghetti Squash Casserole

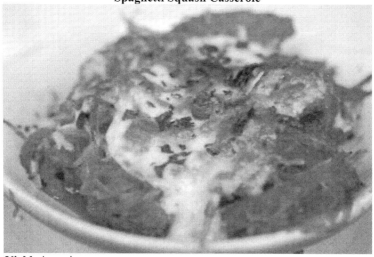

Yield: 4 servings
Ingredients:
1 spaghetti squash
4 large eggs
1 cup sliced onions
½ cup tomatoes, diced
¼ cup Kalamata olives, diced
3 oz salami, finely sliced
4 tbsp bacon fat
2 cloves garlic, minced
Handful of parsley, roughly chopped
Black pepper and sea salt, to taste
Method:
1. Preheat the oven to 400 degrees F.
2. Take the large spaghetti squash and cut it in half, lengthwise. Remove the seeds. Place the two halves on a baking sheet with their cut sides facing up.
3. Spread one tablespoon of bacon fat over the top of each squash. Then sprinkle the black pepper and salt over the squash. Place in the oven for 45 minutes.
4. As the squash bakes, place a skillet over low heat and melt the remaining bacon fat. Then toss in the garlic, onions, and some black pepper and salt.
5. When the onions caramelize, pour in the salami and tomatoes. Sauté over medium heat for 10 more minutes and then toss in the olives.
6. When the squash has baked, remove the two halves from the oven. Scrape out their flesh using a fork. Add the spaghetti squash to the mixture in the skillet.
7. Crack the eggs over the mixture and mix slightly.
8. Pour the mixture into a baking pan and place it inside the oven. Bake until the egg's whites have cooked through.

9. Remove from oven and sprinkle the parsley over the casserole.
10. Serve and enjoy!

Nutritional Values Per Serving:
- Calories – 334
- Fat – 23 g
- Protein – 15 g
- Fiber – 3.8 g
- Net carbs – 13 g

Herb Dumplings With Braised Beef Stew

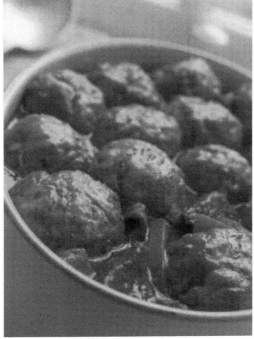

Yield: 6 servings (1 serving is stew plus 2 dumplings)
Ingredients:
For The Stew:
2 lbs braising steak
1 medium carrot
2 cups beef bone broth
1 medium onion, chopped
2 cloves garlic, minced
½ cup dry red wine
7 oz Hokkaido pumpkin
2 tbsp ghee
3 bay leaves
2 tbsp tomato puree
3 sprigs fresh rosemary

¼ tsp black pepper
Salt, to taste
For The Dumplings:
1 cup boiling water
1 large egg
3 large egg whites
½ cup almond flour
1 oz sesame seed flour
1.1 oz coconut flour
1 ½ tsp baking powder (gluten free)
2 ½ tbsp psyllium husk powder
1 tbsp thyme
1 tbsp chopped rosemary
¼ tsp sea salt
For The Topping:
Fresh parsley
A pinch of black pepper
½ a lemon

Method:

1. Preheat the oven to 320 degrees F.
2. Place a large pan over medium heat and melt one tablespoon of ghee. Cook the meat for five minutes and make sure that you stir regularly. Once the meat turns lightly brown, turn the heat off and set the pan aside.
3. Peel the carrots, pumpkin, and onion and chop them into one-inch chunks.
4. Take another large pan and heat the remaining ghee. Cook the vegetables over medium heat as you stir frequently to prevent them from sticking to the bottom. This should take 10 minutes.
5. Add the tomato puree, beef, chopped garlic, bay leaves, and rosemary. Sauté them for two minutes.
6. Pour the wine into the pan and lower the heat. Let it simmer for about five minutes. Then pour in the beef bone broth and add the black pepper and salt. Bring to boil.
7. Warm up a casserole dish by placing it in the oven and then pour the stew into the dish. Cover the casserole dish with a lid and roast for three hours.
8. Once the beef has become tender and all the juices form a thick soup, take the dish out of the oven.
9. Turn up the oven to 350 degrees F.
10. To make dumplings, follow the same instructions as those used when making the *Almond and Sesame Bread* in Day 2 of the meal plan. Once you have mixed all the ingredients together with a mixer, use the dough to form 12 dumplings. Keep the size of the dumplings about one inch in diameter.
11. Get a cupcake tin and grease it with some ghee to prevent the dough from sticking. Place each dumpling in a cupcake well and put the tin in the oven. Bake for about 25 minutes and remove the cupcake tin. Turn

the dumplings over using a spoon and then return the cupcake tin into the oven for another five minutes.

12. If the stew has cooled slightly, put the casserole dish back into the oven to warm it up. Once the stew is hot, remove the casserole dish from the oven and toss the dumplings into the beef stew.

13. Serve the beef stew and dumplings topped with fresh parsley, black pepper, and lemon juice. You can also serve the dish with mashed cauliflower. (This one is also great to make a big batch and portion out for a whole weeks worth of lunches)

Nutritional Values Per Serving:
- Calories – 599
- Fat – 41.8 g
- Protein – 39.8 g
- Net carbs – 8.5 g
- Fiber – 6.7 g

Pork, Cheese, And Spinach Wraps

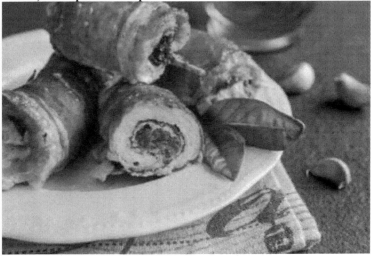

Yield: 4 servings
Ingredients:

2 oz spinach
3 oz feta cheese, crumbled
14 slices bacon
16 oz pork loin
1 medium onion, chopped
½ tsp garlic powder

¾ tsp liquid smoke
½ tsp dried rosemary
2 cloves garlic, minced
1 tbsp olive oil
½ tsp dried thyme
Salt and pepper, to taste

Method:
1. Preheat the oven to 350 degrees F.
2. Pound the pork loin. Cut the pork loin into slices. Then cut the sides of a Ziploc bag, open it up, and place the pork in between the two pieces of plastic. Use a

meat hammer to pound the pork until it forms thin, ¾-inch layers. Massage the pounded pork so that it forms a uniform or flat layer. You should end up with a rectangular block of meat.

3. Take a frying pan and heat the olive oil over high heat. Sauté the onions until soft and then add the garlic. Cook for about one minute.

4. Chop the spinach roughly into small pieces. When the garlic is ready, sauté the spinach for one minute before adding the crumbled feta cheese. Stir the mixture well.

5. Pour half a teaspoon of the liquid smoke, the thyme, and the rosemary into the pan. The leftover liquid smoke will be used later on.

6. Arrange the bacon slices in layers with the edges overlapping one another. Make sure that the layers of bacon are the same length as the block of pork.

7. Place the rectangular block of pounded pork on the bacon slices. Use the remaining ¼ teaspoon of liquid smoke to season the pork. Then sprinkle the salt, pepper, and garlic powder over the meat and rub all the seasoning into the pork.

8. Take the spinach and cheese mixture from the pan and use a spoon to spread it all over the block of pork. Just make sure not to spread it too close to the edges.

9. Wrap the bacon slices around the block of pork and roll it well to make sure the pork is evenly covered by the bacon. To keep the bacon slices in place, use toothpicks to hold the edges.

10. Put the bacon-wrapped pork loin in the oven and roast it for about 75 minutes.

11. Remove the pork from the oven and set aside to cool.

12. Slice the pork into cutlets and serve.

Nutritional Values Per Serving:
- Calories - 606
- Fat – 52 g
- Protein – 30 g
- Net carbs – 3 g
- Fiber – 3 g

Creamy Tuscan Chicken Cutlets

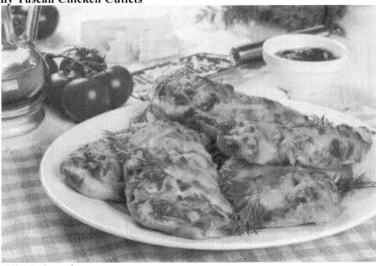

Yield: 6 servings
Ingredients:
3 chicken breasts
4 oz pork rinds
1 large egg
1 cup mozzarella cheese, shredded
½ cup parmesan cheese, shredded
1 cup tomato sauce
¼ cup flaxseed meal
2 tbsp paprika
1 ½ tsp chicken broth
1 ½ tsp oregano
½ tsp minced garlic
½ tsp garlic powder
¼ tsp red pepper flakes
½ cup olive oil
Salt and black pepper
Method:
1. Preheat the oven to 400 degrees F.
2. Place the parmesan cheese, pork rinds, flaxseed meal, paprika, minced garlic, and pepper flakes into a food processor. Combine the ingredients well. This mixture will be used for coating the chicken.
3. Slice the chicken breasts into cutlets and season with some salt and black pepper.
4. Take a large mixing bowl and crack the egg into it. Pour in the chicken broth and whisk them together thoroughly.
5. Take a sauce pan and pour in the tomato sauce, ¼ cup of olive oil, garlic powder, oregano, salt, and black pepper. Whisk the ingredients well.

Place the sauce pan over medium heat and cook for 20 minutes to form a thick sauce.

6. Take a chicken cutlet and dip it into the egg mixture. Then dip the cutlet into the pork rinds mixture to form an even coating around the chicken. Set the cutlet aside on foil paper and repeat the process for all the cutlets.
7. Heat the remaining olive oil in a pan and cook the cutlets. You may have to do this in batches if your pan is not large enough.
8. When the cutlets are ready, put them in a casserole dish and pour the sauce over the chicken. Sprinkle the shreds of mozzarella over the dish.
9. Put the casserole dish in the oven for 10 minutes and let the cheese melt.
10. Serve and enjoy!

Nutritional Values Per Serving:
- Calories – 498
- Fat – 31 g
- Protein – 46.5 g
- Net carbs – 2.6 g

Pork Chops With Mushroom Sauce

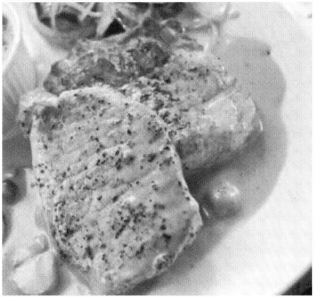

Yield: 4 servings
Ingredients:
4 6-oz pork chops
6 oz mushrooms, sliced
½ cup whipping cream
1 small onion
1 tbsp paprika
1 tbsp fresh parsley, chopped

1 tbsp butter
2 tbsp coconut oil
¼ tsp Xanthan gum
¼ tsp cayenne pepper
1 tsp black pepper
1 tsp salt
1 tsp garlic powder

Method:

1. Place the pork chops under some running water and rinse them. Use a paper towel to dry them and set them aside on a tray.
2. Mix the salt, black pepper, cayenne pepper, paprika, and garlic powder in a small mixing bowl.
3. Take one tablespoon of the spice mixture and sprinkle all over the pork chops. Rub the spices all over the pork chops, making sure that both sides get an even coating. Keep the leftover spices for later use.
4. Place a saucepan on medium heat and pour the coconut oil. Sauté the pork chops for about three minutes on each side until they turn brown. Remove the pork chops and set aside on a plate.
5. Place the sliced mushrooms and onions in the saucepan and then add the pork chops. Cover the pan tightly with a lid and raise the heat. Cook for 25 minutes. Then remove the pork chops and put them on a plate. Don't remove the liquid at the bottom of the pan.
6. Pour the whipping cream, butter, and leftover spice mixture into the hot liquid in the saucepan. Reduce the heat to low setting and whisk the mixture together. Cover the saucepan and let the mixture simmer for about five minutes to form a thick, buttery mushroom sauce.
7. Turn off the heat and pour in the Xanthan gum to thicken the sauce. The sauce will thicken further as it cools.
8. Dress the pork chops with some parsley and mushroom sauce and serve.

Nutritional Values Per Serving:

- Calories – 482
- Fat – 32 g
- Protein – 14.8 g
- Net carbs – 4 g

Stir Fried Beef And Vegetables

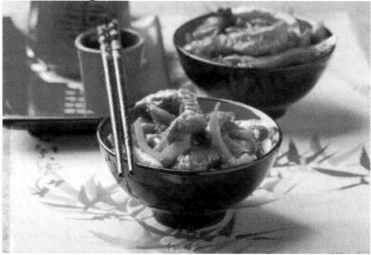

Yield: 4 servings
Ingredients:
1 lb beef steak
1 medium red pepper
2 medium jalapeno peppers
1 clove garlic, minced
1 tbsp oyster sauce
½ tbsp red pepper flakes
1 tbsp rice vinegar
1 tbsp coconut flour
1 tbsp coconut oil
1 tbsp sriracha
4 tbsp soy sauce
1 tbsp minced ginger
1 tbsp roasted sesame seeds
1 tbsp sesame oil
6 drops liquid Stevia
Cooking oil
Method:
1. Slice the beef steak into ¼-inch thick strips.
2. Thinly slice the jalapeno and red peppers.
3. Take a large skillet and pour in the coconut oil. Place the skillet over medium heat. When the oil becomes hot, fry the red pepper slices, minced garlic, and minced ginger. When they start to produce a scent, add the oyster sauce, soy sauce, sesame oil, sriracha, rice vinegar, and Stevia. Mix well using a whisk for two minutes. Then add the sesame seeds and pepper flakes. Stir well.

4. Meanwhile, take a large pot and place it over high heat. Pour in one inch of the cooking oil and fry the beef strips. Make sure that you don't cook too many at once. When one side of the beef has turned dark brown, flip over to the other side.

5. When all the beef strips are cooked, remove them and place them on a plate with a paper towel. This is to soak up excess oil.

6. Place the fried beef into the large skillet containing the spicy sauce. Stir well and cook for two minutes. Let the beef strips soak up the flavor of the sauce.

7. Place the beef strips in serving bowls and garnish with the jalapeno and red pepper slices.

8. Serve and enjoy!

Nutritional Values Per Serving:

- Calories – 406
- Fat – 31g
- Protein – 24 g
- Net carbs – 4.2 g

Creamy Asparagus Soup

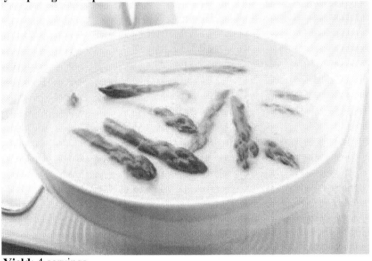

Yield: 4 servings
Ingredients:
1.1 lbs fresh asparagus spears
1 clove garlic, chopped
2 tbsp ghee
1 brown onion, chopped
1 tsp extra virgin olive oil
¾ cup coconut cream
4 cups chicken bone broth
Sea salt and pepper, to taste

Method:

1. Chop off the woody and tough stems of the asparagus. Then peel the remaining stem using a vegetable peeler.
2. Place a saucepan over medium heat and melt the butter. Sauté the onions and garlic for about two minutes.
3. Cut the asparagus into pieces and toss them into the saucepan. Add the chicken broth and increase the heat from medium to high setting. Let the asparagus cook until it becomes soft but not soggy.
4. Remove the saucepan from the heat and blend the mixture using an immersion blender. The mixture should acquire a smooth consistency.
5. To make the consistency of the soup more silky and smooth, strain it using a fine mesh sieve.
6. Pour the strained soup back into the saucepan. Add salt, pepper, and coconut cream.
7. Heat the soup until it becomes hot, but don't let it boil.
8. Drizzle the olive oil over the soup and serve. You can also allow the soup to cool and store in the refrigerator for a maximum of four days.

Nutritional Values Per Serving:

- Calories – 350
- Fat – 32.3 g
- Protein – 8.7 g
- Net carbs – 4.8 g
- Fiber – 3 g

Keto Kale And Pork Chops

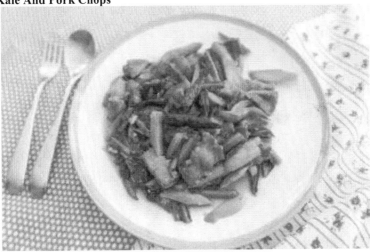

Yield: 4 servings
Ingredients:
7.1 oz kale leaves
6 oz bonless pork chops
1 jalapeno

2 tbsp apple cider vinegar
1 clove garlic, minced
2tbsp. Soy Sauce
Pink Himalayan salt or sea salt, to taste
Method:
1. Wash the kale leaves and pat them dry using paper towels.
2. Break off the stems and chop the leaves.
3. Slice the pork chops into ½-inch pieces.
4. Slice the jalapeno into strips.
5. Place a large skillet over high heat and cook the pork chops until they turn golden brown and crispy.
6. Add the jalapeno slices and minced garlic into the skillet. Sauté for 30 seconds.
7. Pour the chopped kale leaves into the skillet. Cook until the kale starts to wilt.
8. Pour in the apple cider vinegar and soy sauce and cook for 10 more minutes until the kale softens. Then season with the salt and serve.

Nutritional Values Per Serving:
- Calories – 165
- Fat – 15.2 g
- Protein – 3.7 g
- Net carbs – 2.2 g
- Fiber – 1.1 g

Cheesy Spinach Stuffed Mushroom Caps

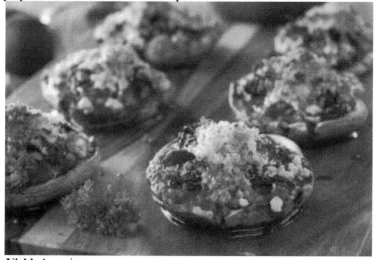

Yield: 4 servings
Ingredients:
1.5 lbs Portobello mushrooms
10 oz fresh spinach
¼ cup ricotta

½ cup parmesan, grated
¼ cup cheddar cheese, grated
3.5 oz goat cheese
1 cup cream cheese
2 tbsp butter
1/8 tsp dried Italian herbs
2 tbsp red bell pepper, diced
½ small red onion, chopped
½ tsp garlic, minced

Method:

1. Preheat the oven to 355 degrees F.
2. Remove the stems and gills of the mushrooms. Use a paper towel to thoroughly dry the mushroom caps.
3. Melt the butter in a pan and pour in a small bowl. Use a brush to smear the melted butter over the mushroom caps. Make sure you brush both the inside and outside.
4. Line a baking tray with parchment paper and place the mushroom caps on the tray.
5. Finely chop the spinach leaves and red onion. Place them in a large bowl and add the ricotta, parmesan, cream cheese, goat cheese, and minced garlic. Mix the ingredients well.
6. Use a spoon to scoop the mixture into the mushroom caps. Don't be afraid to fill the mushroom caps all the way to the top and then some. The mixture will not melt and run in the oven.
7. Top the mixture with the diced red peppers and grated cheddar cheese.
8. Place the baking tray in the oven for 20 minutes. The mushroom topping should turn slightly brown and appear bubbly.
9. Garnish with some fresh herbs and serve. If anything is left over, you can use it as stuffing for chicken breasts.

Nutritional Values Per Serving:

- Calories – 432
- Fat – 36.8 g
- Protein – 22.8 g
- Net carbs – 8.9 g
- Fiber - 4.6 g

Goat Cheese Burgers

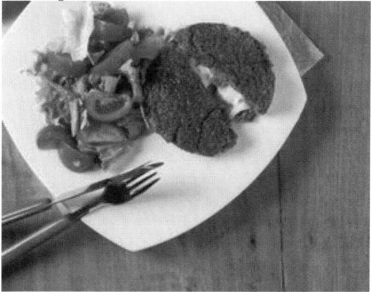

Yield: 2 burgers/servings
Ingredients:
14.1 oz ground beef
3 tbsp duck fat
4.5 oz soft goat cheese
Salt, to taste
Method:
1. Preheat the oven to 400 degrees F.
2. Put the cheese in the freezer for about half an hour. Though this step is optional, it helps to stop the cheese from oozing out when the burgers are being cooked.
3. Remove the cheese and ground beef from the freezer. Use your hands to make two meat patties. Take one piece of goat cheese and place it in the centre of the first patty. Then wrap the meat around the cheese to form a ball. Do the same for the other patty. It is important to make sure that the meat totally covers the cheese so that it won't ooze out.
4. Place an ovenproof skillet over high heat and melt the remaining duck fat. Cook the burgers for one minute, flip them over, and cook the other side. Season with the salt.
5. Put the skillet in the oven and bake the burgers for about eight minutes. Remove the skillet and set aside for five minutes.
6. Serve the burgers with vegetable salad.

Nutritional Values Per Serving:
Calories – 857
Fat – 69 g
Protein – 48.9 g

Net carbs – 7.3 g
Fiber – 1.4 g

Mediterranean Chicken And Veggie Delight

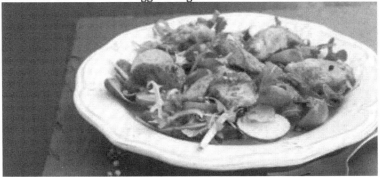

Yield: 4 servings
Ingredients:
1 ½ lbs chicken breast
1.4 oz spinach
1 cup cherry tomatoes
½ cup yellow onion, diced
2 tbsp extra virgin olive oil
1 ½ tbsp Greek seasoning
½ lemon, sliced
2 tbsp lemon juice
4 garlic cloves, minced
1.2 oz Kalamata olives
8 oz white button mushrooms, sliced
14 oz artichoke hearts
Salt, to taste
For Topping:
4 tbsp extra virgin olive oil
2 tbsp basil, chopped
Method:
1. Dice the onion, mince the garlic, slice the mushrooms, and slice the lemon.
2. Slice the chicken breasts into 1-inch cubes.
3. Place a large pan over medium-high heat and pour in the olive oil. Add the chicken and season with the Greek seasoning and salt. (*If you do not have Greek seasoning, you can make your own by combining ½ teaspoon dried mint, ½ teaspoon dried thyme, 1 teaspoon dried oregano, ¼ teaspoon garlic powder, ½ teaspoon onion powder, ¼ teaspoon dried marjoram, and ½ teaspoon dried basil.*)
4. Cook the chicken for five minutes until the chicken pieces turn golden. Then place the chicken on a plate.

5. Use the same pan to cook the onions and garlic for about a minute. When the onions become fragrant, add the olives, mushrooms, artichokes, tomatoes, lemon slices, and lemon juice. Cook for five minutes until the mushrooms become soft.
6. Add the chicken pieces to the vegetable mix and toss the mixture. Add the spinach and cook until they wilt.
7. Chop the basil and sprinkle over the chicken. Garnish with slices of lemon and drizzle the olive oil.
8. Turn off the heat and serve while hot.

Nutritional Values Per Serving:
- Calories – 463
- Fat – 27.5 g
- Protein – 40.9 g
- Net carbs – 6.9 g
- Fiber – 7.6 g

Focaccia Kale Salad

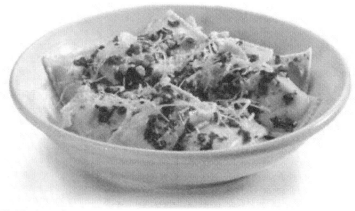

Yield: 4 servings
Ingredients:
For The Salad:
1 batch (Keto Focaccia bread from Breakfast Section)
¼ cup parmesan, shaved
3 tbsp. olive oil
½ lb kale leaves, finely chopped
½ tsp garlic powder
Salt, to taste
For The Dressing:
3 tbsp parmesan cheese, grated
3 cloves garlic, minced
¾ cup mayonnaise
2 tsp Dijon mustard
1 tbsp anchovy paste

½ lemon
2 tsp Worcestershire sauce
Method:
1. Preheat the oven to 375 degrees F.
2. Make the Focaccia bread using the recipe provided on Day 10 of the Breakfast meal plan. There's no need for any of the toppings.
3. Once you have baked the Focaccia bread, slice the loaf into cubes the size of croutons. Place the cubes in a mixing bowl and toss with the salt, olive oil, and garlic powder.
4. Line a baking pan with parchment paper and arrange the Focaccia cubes on the baking sheet.
5. Place the baking tray in the oven for 15 minutes. Flip the cubes to make sure they become crisp.
6. Take all the ingredients for making the dressing and place them in a glass jar. Shake the jar well until all the ingredients combine. Then place the jar in the refrigerator.
7. When the dressing has chilled, use it to toss the chopped kale leaves.
8. Remove the croutons and add them to the dressed kale. Then top with the shaved parmesan and serve.

Nutritional Values Per Serving:
- Calories – 398
- Fat – 36.6 g
- Protein – 10.5 g
- Net carbs – 4.8 g
- Fiber – 3.6 g

Spinach, Bacon, And Mushroom Frittata

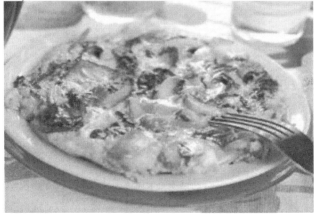

Yield: 6 servings
Ingredients:
4 Baby Bella mushrooms
8 slices bacon
8 large eggs
2 cups spinach, chopped

¼ cup parmesan cheese, grated
¼ cup heavy cream
4 oz fresh mozzarella, cubed
2 oz goat cheese, grated
1 tbsp coconut oil
¼ cup sundried tomatoes, chopped
Salt and ground black pepper, to taste
Method:
1. Preheat your oven to 350 degrees F.
2. Roughly chop the slices of bacon and mushrooms, making sure to remove the mushroom stems before chopping.
3. Place an oven-proof skillet over medium heat and pour in the coconut oil. When the oil becomes hot, add the bacon.
4. When the bacon pieces begin to turn slightly brown, add the dried tomatoes and spinach pieces. Stir well. As the veggies and bacon are cooking, start preparing your egg mixture.
5. Take a large mixing bowl and crack the eggs into it. Add the grated parmesan cheese, heavy cream, and black pepper. Mix the ingredients thoroughly to ensure a smooth consistency.
6. Take the chopped mushrooms and toss them into the skillet containing the bacon and vegetables. Stir the mixture well and leave for a while. This is to allow the mushrooms to soak up the fat in the pan.
7. Take the chopped mozzarella cubes and toss them into the skillet. Then pour the egg mixture over all the ingredients in the skillet. Make sure that you distribute the egg mixture uniformly.
8. Use a wooden ladle to mix the ingredients slowly. Make sure that the egg reaches the bottom of the pan and goes all around the mushrooms, bacon, and tomatoes.
9. Take the grated goat cheese and sprinkle it over the top of the frittata. Place the skillet into the oven and leave for about 10 minutes. The top of the frittata should turn a golden-brown color.
10. Take the skillet out and allow it to cool for about one minute.
11. Use a spoon to gently lift the edges of the frittata from the skillet. This is to make sure that it will be easy to remove.
12. Place some parchment paper on a baking sheet, and then flip the skillet over onto the paper.
13. Flip the frittata over using a cutting board.
14. Slice into wedges and serve. (This is great for Lunch at home, or breakfast)

Nutritional Values Per Serving:
*   Calories – 434
*   Fat – 37 g
*   Protein – 23.2 g
*   Net carbs – 4.76 g
*   Fiber – 0.73 g

Lemon-Stuffed Grilled Trout

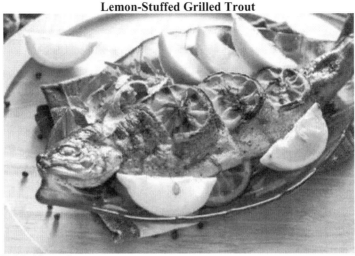

Yield: 10 servings
Ingredients:
For The Trout:
7.7 lbs whole trout
2.7 oz ghee
4 small onions
2 whole lemons
Bunch of arugula salad leaves
Salt and pepper, to taste
For The Tarragon Sauce:
1 tbsp white wine vinegar
4.5 oz melted butter
1 tbsp tarragon, chopped
3 egg yolks
Sea salt and black pepper, to taste
Method:
1. Preheat the oven to 465 degrees F.
2. Peel the onions and slice each in half.
3. Slice each lemon in half. Set two halves aside and slice the other two halves into thin wedges or slices. Cut the ghee into slices.
4. Take the whole trout and use a sharp knife to make a number of slashes on both sides of the fish. Sprinkle the black pepper and salt into the cavities and then place the lemon wedges and onion slices into the spaces. Push the slices of ghee into the slashes as well.
5. Use kitchen twine to tie the trout at intervals so that the stuffing doesn't fall out. Place the stuffed trout on a rack and grill for 15 minutes on each side.
6. Remove the grilled trout and set it aside to cool slightly.
7. Slice the remaining lemon pieces into wedges. Then place the arugula leaves and lemon wedges on a platter.

8. Carefully place the trout on top of the arugula leaves and then remove the kitchen twine.
9. Place the vinegar and egg yolks into a blender and mix them until a creamy liquid is produced. Then add the melted butter in intervals as the blender continues to mix. When the sauce becomes thick, add the chopped tarragon and mix for a few more seconds. Add salt and black pepper, to taste.
10. Serve and enjoy! (Great for a fancy lunch or Brunch on the weekend)

Nutritional Values Per Serving:
- Calories – 428
- Fat – 28.2 g
- Protein – 39.2 g
- Net carbs – 2.1 g
- Fiber – 0.5 g

Creamy Cauliflower Masala

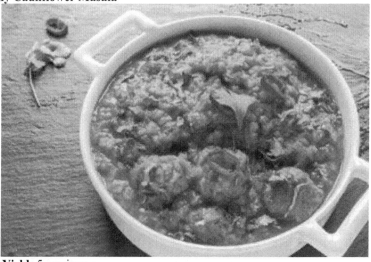

Yield: 5 servings
Ingredients:
For The Cauliflower:
1.4 lbs cauliflower, chopped into florets
½ tsp cayenne pepper
1 tsp garam masala
1 tsp ground cumin
1 tbsp olive oil
1 large red bell pepper, chopped
½ tsp salt
For The Sauce:
12.7 oz tomatoes, crushed
4 tbsp virgin coconut oil
¼ cup cilantro, minced

½ white onion, sliced
½ cup heavy whipping cream
1 tbsp ginger, minced
2 cloves garlic, minced
½ cup water
½ tsp cayenne pepper
1 tbsp garam masala
1 tsp ground cumin
1 ½ tsp paprika
Salt, to taste

Method:
1. Preheat the oven to 425 degrees F.
2. Place the chopped florets in a large bowl and toss with the spices and olive oil.
3. Line a baking sheet with some foil and lay the florets on the sheet. Place the baking sheet in the oven and bake the florets for half an hour.
4. Start preparing the sauce 15 minutes before removing the florets from the oven. Take a large skillet and place it over medium-high heat. Melt the butter and cook the onions, ginger, and garlic for about five minutes. Make sure that the onions start to caramelize.
5. Add the rest of the spices for the sauce into the skillet and cook for about 30 seconds. Then add the tomatoes, heavy cream, and water. Stir occasionally for 10 minutes until the sauce begins to simmer.
6. The cauliflower should be ready by now. Pour the baked cauliflower into the skillet and stir well to ensure a good mix.
7. Top with the minced cilantro and chopped red bell peppers.
8. Serve and enjoy!

Nutritional Values Per Serving:
- Calories – 249
- Fat – 21.1 g
- Protein – 4.7 g
- Net carbs – 9.9 g
- Fiber – 4.9 g

Brined Fried Chicken Drumsticks

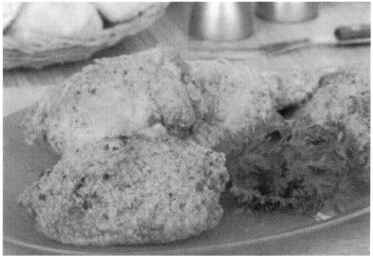

Yield: 6 servings
Ingredients:
3.5 lbs chicken drumsticks
4 cups almond milk
2.2 oz pork rinds
4 tbsp lemon juice
¼ cup coconut flour
2 tbsp sea salt
1 tsp onion powder
2 tsp ground black pepper
1 tsp garlic powder
2 tsp dried oregano
2 tsp smoked paprika
Olive oil for cooking
Method:
1. Preheat the oven to 360 degrees F.
2. Take a mixing bowl and pour in the almond milk, salt, lemon juice, one teaspoon of dried oregano, and one teaspoon of black pepper. Mix well.
3. Dip the chicken drumsticks into the brine mixture for 90 minutes. You can also leave them overnight for extra flavor.
4. Pour all the remaining ingredients into a food processor, with the exception of the olive oil. Mix the ingredients to create a floury, crumb-like mixture.
5. Pour the crumby mixture onto a tray. Take one drumstick at a time out of the brine liquid and roll it in the crumbs. Make sure that the chicken is coated evenly on all sides. Place the coated drumstick on a lined baking tray and repeat the process for all the other drumsticks.

6. When all the pieces have been coated, place the lined baking tray in the oven and bake for about 25 minutes. Remove the tray from the oven and spray/drizzle the olive oil over the chicken pieces. Then return the tray into the oven and bake for another 20 minutes.
7. Serve and enjoy!

Nutritional Values Per Serving:
- Calories – 314
- Fat – 17.1 g
- Protein – 31.6 g
- Net carbs – 2 g
- Fiber – 1.7 g

Extra Krispy Chicken Wings With Sauce

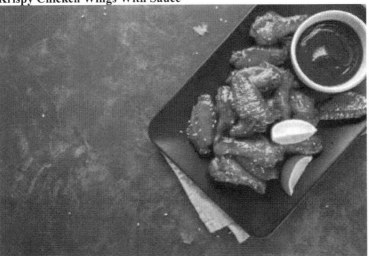

Yield: 8 servings
Ingredients:
24 chicken wings
2 tbsp duck fat, melted
2 tbsp gluten-free baking powder
1 tsp salt
For The Sauce:
¼ cup lime juice
1 tbsp fish sauce
Liquid Stevia to taste
¼ cup coconut aminos
4 cloves garlic, minced
1 small chili pepper
1 tbsp ginger, finely grated
Method:
1. Preheat the oven to 250 degrees F.
2. Adjust the racks in the oven to be at the upper-middle and lower-middle positions. Get a deep baking tray and line it with baking foil. Then set a rack on top of the foil.

3. Cut the chicken wings at the joints using a sharp knife. This will produce three pieces for every wing. Use a paper towel to dry the chicken wings.
4. Remove the wingtips and set them aside in the freezer. You will not need them in this particular recipe, but you can use them to make your favorite chicken broth recipe.
5. Take the remaining pieces of chicken wings and place them inside a bowl and add the salt and baking powder. Toss the wings to get an even coating.
6. Arrange the chicken wings on the rack on top of the foil. Make sure that the side of the wing with the skin is facing up.
7. Use a brush to apply the melted ghee all over the chicken wings.
8. Place the baking tray on the lower rack of the oven and bake for half an hour. This will render the fat. Then move the tray onto the upper rack to make the chicken crispy. Raise the temperature to 425 degrees F and bake for 45 minutes.
9. Meanwhile, make the sauce. Take a saucepan and pour in all the ingredients for the sauce. Chop the pepper into small pieces before adding to the mixture. Mix well and then place the saucepan over medium-low heat. Bring to a boil gradually and cook for 10 minutes. The sauce should turn brown and thick.
10. When the chicken wings are evenly cooked, take the tray out of the oven and set it aside. Allow the wings to cool for five minutes.
11. Serve the chicken wings with the sauce as a dip rather than a topping. If the wings are coated in sauce, they will quickly lose their crispiness.

Nutritional Values Per Serving:
- Calories – 335
- Fat – 23.4 g
- Protein – 22.8 g
- Net carbs – 3.1 g
- Fiber – 7.6 g

Chapter Six: Dinner Recipes

The following recipes offer a wide range of variety and complexity. I wanted to give you options here so there will be a great dinner recipe suitable for any occasion and any amount of available cooking time. You will be spoiled for choices of delicious recipes here and if you're like me, as soon as you read them, you're going to want to run to the kitchen to start trying them out.

Keto Pork Lettuce Wraps

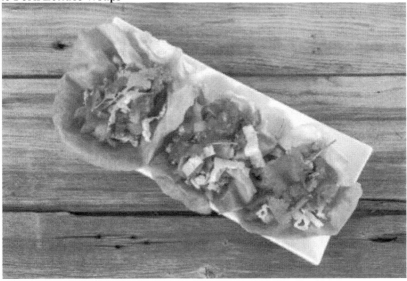

Yield: 3 servings
Ingredients:
1 medium red bell pepper
6 pork ribs
¼ medium yellow onion
2 cloves garlic, minced
1 tbsp. fresh ginger, minced
6 leaves lettuce
Method:
1. Use a sharp knife to cut and separate the pork ribs. Then use your hands to strip the meat from the bones. Use the knife to slice the meat into bite-sized shreds.
2. Slice the onion and red bell pepper into thin strips. Saute with the minced garlic and ginger in a medium skillet over medium heat until fragrant and the peppers and onions start to soften slightly.
3. Place the lettuce leaves on a serving tray and add the shredded pork on top. Then add the onion and pepper mixture on top.
4. Roll the lettuce to cover the filling. If you prefer, you can top with some chili sauce.
5. Serve and enjoy!
Nutritional Values Per Serving:
- Calories – 338
- Fat – 25.6 g
- Protein – 24 g
- Net carbs – 2.5 g

Chorizo Stuffed Spaghetti Squash

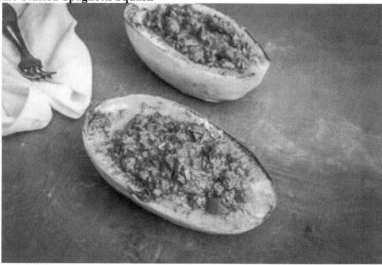

Yield: 4 servings
Ingredients:
1 lb Mexican chorizo
2 small spaghetti squashes
2 cups canned tomatoes
1 small brown onion, chopped
2 tbsp lard
1 cup shredded cheddar cheese
Parsley for topping
Freshly ground black pepper and salt

Method:

1. Preheat the oven to 400 degrees F.
2. Slice the squashes in half and use a spoon to scoop out the seeds. The seeds can either be thrown away or stored for later use as a snack (roasted squash seeds).
3. Melt the lard in a pan. Use a brush to smear the melted lard over the inside of the squashes. Save some of the lard for later and then season the squashes with salt.
4. Place the squashes on a baking tray and bake in the oven for about 30 minutes. Use a fork to check whether the squashes are cooked. The size of the squash will determine how long it takes to cook.
5. As the squashes are baking, place a large pan over medium heat and pour in the leftover lard. Sauté the onions until they turn light brown.
6. Pour the chorizo into the pan and cook for five minutes. When the chorizo turns brown, add the tomatoes, salt, and black pepper. Cook for about two minutes.

7. Grate the cheddar cheese and sprinkle it over the chorizo (save some of the cheese for topping). Stir the mixture well and when ready, remove the pan from the heat.
8. When the squashes are ready, remove them from the oven. Use the chorizo mixture to fill the squash halves.
9. Use the leftover grated cheese as topping and place the squash halves under a broiler for five minutes. When the cheese has melted and become slightly crispy, remove the squashes.
10. Top with chopped parsley and serve immediately.

Nutritional Values Per Serving:
- Calories – 548
- Fat – 40.3 g
- Protein – 27 g
- Net carbs – 16.4 g
- Fiber – 5.3 g

Sweet And Spicy Pork Roast

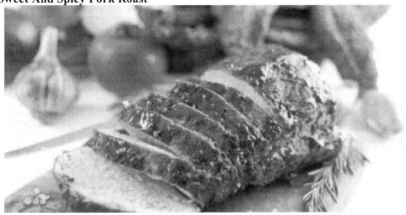

Yield: 10 servings
Ingredients:
4.4 lbs pork loin roast
1 tbsp fresh ginger, grated
2 tsp orange zest
4 tbsp granulated Erythritol
4 cloves garlic, minced
2 tbsp extra virgin olive oil
½ tsp red chili flakes
2 tbsp melted ghee
¼ tsp ground cloves
1 ½ tsp salt
¼ tsp black pepper

Method:

1. Take a small mixing bowl and pour in the grated ginger, granulated Erythritol, minced garlic, orange zest, chili flakes, salt, black pepper, and ground cloves. Mix all the ingredients well.
2. Pour in the olive oil and melted ghee. Use a spoon to mix well.
3. Put the pork on a piece of plastic wrap and rub the spices all over it. Cover the pork with the wrap and tie it with some kitchen twine to hold it together.
4. Place the pork on a pan and put it in the fridge overnight. This will help the pork absorb all the spicy flavors.
5. Take the pork out of the fridge and let it sit for an hour at room temperature. In the meantime, preheat the oven to 400 degrees F.
6. Roast the pork in the oven for about 15 minutes.
7. Lower the heat to 320 degrees F and continue baking for two more hours. Use an Instant-Read thermometer to check the temperature of the pork, which should be between 135 to 140 degrees F.
8. Remove the pork roast and set it aside for 15 minutes.
9. Cut the pork into slices and serve with cauliflower mash or Brussels sprouts.

Nutritional Values Per Serving:
- Calories – 451
- Fat – 30.9 g
- Protein – 39.5 g
- Net carbs – 0.7 g
- Fiber – 0.2 g

Keto Beef Short Ribs

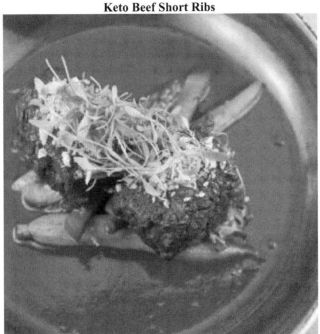

Yield: 4 servings
Ingredients:
8 beef short ribs
2 celery stalks, chopped
2 cups spinach, pre-cooked
2 tbsp coconut oil
3 cloves garlic, chopped
¾ cup tomato sauce
2 tbsp ghee
8 oz fresh tomatoes
1 cup dry white wine
Salt and pepper, to taste
Method:
1. Unpack the short ribs and cut them up into eight big pieces of the same size. Use the salt and pepper to generously season the ribs.
2. Place a skillet over medium heat and melt the coconut oil. Sauté the beef ribs until they turn brown all round. Then remove the ribs from the skillet and place them in a crock pot.
3. Deglaze the wine in the skillet and pour in the tomato sauce. Chop the tomatoes into large chunks and toss them into the skillet. Stir the mixture well.
4. Pour the contents of the skillet over the beef ribs in the crock pot. Add all the remaining ingredients into the pot and stir well. Make sure that as you stir the mixture, some of the vegetables end up at the bottom of the crock pot while some are on top of the ribs.

5. Cover the crock pot and cook over high heat for about six hours. It is important that you avoid opening the lid except to turn over the ribs.
6. When ready, garnish with some horseradish gremolata and seasonal vegetables.
7. Serve and enjoy with some Keto bread.

Nutritional Values Per Serving:
- Calories – 512
- Fat – 39.9 g
- Protein – 26.3 g
- Net carbs – 6.1 g
- Fiber – 2.7 g

Breaded Cod Fillet

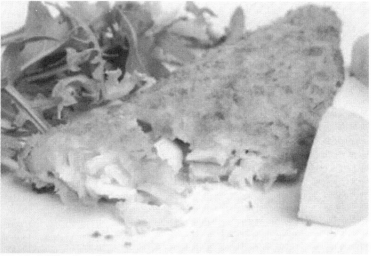

Yield: 4 fillets/servings
Ingredients:
4 cod fillets, skinless
1 large egg
¼ cup ghee
1 cup almond flour
A pinch of ground caraway seeds
4 tbsp flax meal
1 tbsp coconut milk
Salt and pepper, to taste

Method:

1. Take a medium mixing bowl and combine the flax meal and almond flour.
2. Place the cod fillets on a tray and remove the excess moisture using paper towels. Season the fillets on both sides using the ground caraway, salt, and pepper.
3. Take a small bowl and crack the egg into it. Add the coconut milk and a pinch of salt. Beat the mixture using a fork.
4. Dip one of the cod fillets into the egg mixture and then dip it into the bowl containing the flax meal and almond flour. Ensure all sides of the fillet are coated and then shake it gently to get rid of any excess coating. Set the fillet aside and repeat the process for the other three fillets.
5. Place a large pan over medium-high heat and melt the ghee. When the pan becomes hot, fry the breaded fillets until they turn golden brown. Then turn the fillets over and fry the other side. Avoid turning the fish over too soon or the coating will come off.
6. Place the cod fillets on a serving plate and serve with salad.

Nutritional Values Per Serving:

- Calories – 464
- Fat – 33.5 g
- Protein – 35 g
- Net carbs – 5.7 g
- Fiber – 4.4 g

Haddock Fillet Cakes With Mayo Sauce

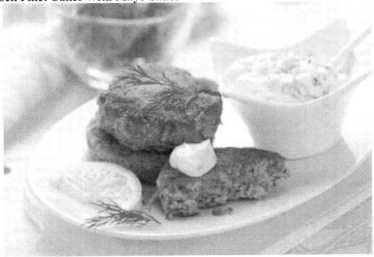

Yield: 18 patties
Ingredients:
1.76 lbs haddock fish fillets, boneless and skinless
2 large eggs
1 large onion, chopped

2 cups cauliflower rice, prepared
4 tbsp flax meal
4 tbsp coconut oil
½ cup parmesan cheese, grated
1 clove garlic, minced
2 tbsp fresh parsley, chopped
1 tsp ground cumin
1 tsp lemon zest
Salt and black pepper, to taste

For The Sauce:
2 cloves garlic, minced
½ cup mayonnaise

Method:

1. Take a large and deep pan and cook the cauliflower rice.
2. Take another small saucepan and place over medium heat. Pour in one tablespoon of coconut oil and sauté the minced garlic for about 30 seconds.
3. Then add the cooked cauliflower rice and some salt. Cook for five minutes and stir occasionally. When ready, remove the pan from the heat and place it aside.
4. Place the fish fillets on a tray and pat them dry using paper towels. Season the fish with salt and pepper.
5. Place a large pan over medium heat and pour in one tablespoon of coconut oil. When the oil becomes hot, cook the fish for about 3 minutes. Flip the fish over using a spatula and cook the other side for another two minutes. The cooking time depends on how thick the fillets are). The fish should be flaky and opaque in color.
6. Remove the fillets from the pan and set aside on a large bowl for five minutes.
7. Place the cooked cauliflower, onions, flax meal, almond flour, lemon zest, chopped parsley, eggs, and ground cumin into the large bowl containing the fillets. Combine the mixture thoroughly. Season the mixture with some salt and pepper and mix well.
8. Make the patties using a ¼ measuring cup. Scoop some of the mixture into the measuring cup and flatten using a spoon. Flip the cup over onto a chopping board to remove the patty from the cup. Reshape the patty using your hands. Follow the same procedure to make the rest of the patties.
9. Place a large frying pan over medium-high heat. Use one tablespoon of coconut oil to fry the first batch of patties for three to five minutes per side. The patties should turn golden. Make sure you don't overfill the pan and avoid flipping the patties too soon or the crust will break. Use a spatula to test whether a patty is ready.
10. To prepare the sauce, mix the mayonnaise and minced garlic.
11. Serve the fish cakes with the sauce and some low-carb salad.

Nutritional Values Per Serving:

- Calories – 449
- Fat – 34.2 g
- Protein – 29.7 g

- Net carbs – 3.1 g
- Fiber – 3.2 g

Salmon Keto Bowl

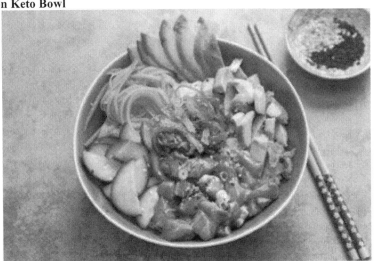

Yield: 2 servings
Ingredients:
For The Salmon:
½ lb salmon, skin and bones removed
1 tbsp sesame seeds
2 tbsp coconut aminos
2 medium green onions, chopped
1 tbsp lime juice
1 tsp coconut vinegar
1 tbsp toasted sesame oil
1 tsp Sriracha sauce
Salt, to taste
For The Cauli-Rice:
2 cups cauliflower riced
¼ tsp salt
1 tbsp coconut vinegar
1 tbsp coconut oil
For The Topping:
1 tbsp coconut oil
1 cup seaweed
1 avocado
1 large cucumber
1 large carrot
Method:

1. Take a large mixing bowl and make a marinade of coconut aminos, lime juice, toasted sesame oil, salt, and vinegar. Mix well.
2. Chop the salmon into bite-sized chunks and place them in a separate mixing bowl.
3. Pour the marinade over the salmon chunks and add the sesame seeds and sriracha. Mix well.
4. Place the bowl in the refrigerator as you make the cauliflower rice.
5. Place a pan over medium-high heat and add the coconut oil. When the oil becomes hot, cook the cauli-rice for five minutes, making sure to stir well to avoid burning the rice.
6. Take a small bowl and mix the salt and vinegar.
7. When the cauli-rice is cooked, pour it into a bowl and add the vinegar mix.
8. Grease a pan with coconut oil and cook the seaweed over medium heat until it turns crisp. This should take about 30 seconds. Add salt, to taste.
9. Cut the avocado in half, remove the seed, and peel it. Cut the avocado into slices. Cut the cucumber into half-slices and chop the carrot into very thin strips.
10. Serve the cauli-rice in two serving bowls and add the chunks of cooked salmon. Top with the seaweed, sliced cucumber, carrot strips, and avocado slices.

Nutritional Values Per Serving:
- Calories – 558
- Fat – 42.4 g
- Protein – 30.3 g
- Net carbs – 8.5 g
- Fiber – 8.8 g

Keto Steak Salad

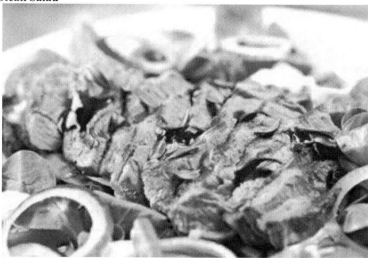

Yield: 2 servings

Ingredients:
For The Steak:
10.6 oz ribeye steaks
1 tbsp ghee
Freshly ground black pepper
Salt
For The Salad:
7.1 oz mixed greens of your choice
1 large red bell pepper, sliced
1 large green pepper, sliced
1tbsp ghee
1 clove garlic, minced
½ cup mozzarella cheese, grated
1 small yellow onion, sliced
Fresh herbs as garnish
Salt and pepper
Method:
1. Set the steak on a tray to thaw for 10 minutes. Use a paper towel to wipe off any excess blood and moisture. Melt one tablespoon of ghee and toss the steak with the oil. Then use salt and pepper to season the meat.
2. Place a cast-iron griddle pan over high heat and fry the steak for four minutes per side. When one side turns brown, flip over.
3. When the steak is cooked, set it aside for five minutes. Place it on parchment paper and fold it up. Then cover it with a kitchen towel. This is to keep all the juices inside.
4. After the five minutes are up, slice the steak into strips.
5. Prepare the veggies by melting the ghee in the cast-iron pan. Slice the peppers and onion and sauté in the pan. Add the minced garlic and grated cheese, and cook for three minutes.
6. Take a serving bowl and assemble the lettuce. Pour in the cooked peppers, onions, and garlic. Then add the steak strips.
7. Serve warm.

Nutritional Values Per Serving:
- Calories – 622
- Fat – 47.1 g
- Protein – 38.1 g
- Net carbs – 8.3 g
- Fiber – 4 g

Baked Sea Bass

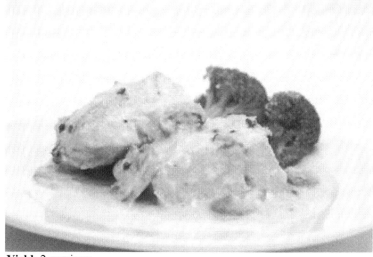

Yield: 2 servings
Ingredients:
10.6 oz sea bass fillets
2.1 oz pesto
1 tbsp lemon juice
1 tbsp coconut oil
Salt, to taste
Method:
1. Preheat the oven to 400 degrees F.
2. Take a baking tray and line it with parchment paper. Set the sea bass fillets in the tray with the skin side facing down.
3. Use the salt and pepper to season the fillets, and then use a brush to smear the coconut oil over the top of the fillets. Pour the lemon juice over the fish.
4. Place the baking tray in the oven and cook for 10 minutes.
5. When ready, remove the tray and top the fillets with pesto. Put the tray back in the oven and cook for another five minutes.
6. Remove the fillets and set aside to cool for five minutes.
7. Serve with roasted broccoli.

Nutritional Values Per Serving:
- Calories – 423
- Fat – 32.9 g
- Protein – 29.3 g
- Net carbs – 1.5 g
- Fiber – 0.7 g

Eggplant Parmesan

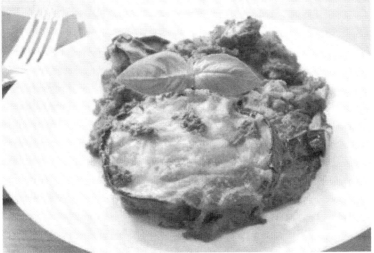

Yield: 4 servings
Ingredients:
1 large egg
1.1 lb eggplant
1 cup parmesan cheese, grated
½ tsp salt
¼ cup coconut oil
1 tsp dried Italian herbs
1 tbsp almond milk
½ cup coconut flour
½ cup almond flour
Salt and pepper, to taste

Method:

1. Chop the eggplant into ¼-inch slices and season each slice with the half teaspoon of salt. Set the slices aside for an hour.
2. Use a paper towel to pat the slices dry to remove any excess moisture.
3. Take a small bowl and crack the egg into it. Add the cream and beat with a fork.
4. Grate the parmesan into a bowl and add the Italian herbs. Mix well.
5. In a different bowl, mix the almond and coconut flour.
6. Take the eggplant slices and dip them in the egg mixture, then the cheese, and finally the flour mix.
7. Place a large pan over medium-high heat and melt the coconut oil. Cook the eggplant slices for three minutes. Do this in batches to prevent overcrowding in the pan.
8. Serve hot.

Nutritional Values Per Serving:
- Calories – 405
- Fat – 31.2 g
- Protein – 16.2 g
- Net carbs – 7.3 g
- Fiber – 7.8 g

Spicy Beef Stroganoff Stew

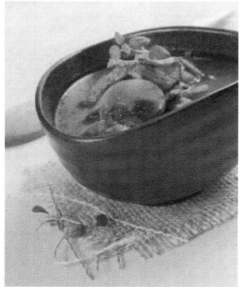

Yield: 6 servings
Ingredients:
2 large sirloin steaks
5 cups chicken bone broth
1.3 lbs brown mushrooms
12.2 oz sour cream
¼ cup ghee
2 cloves garlic, minced
4 tbsp lemon juice
1 medium onion, chopped
1 tbsp Dijon mustard
2 tsp paprika
¼ tsp black pepper
1 tsp salt
Method:
1. Freeze the steaks for 30 minutes to make it easier to slice them into strips.
2. Meanwhile, wash and chop the mushrooms into slices.
3. Slice the steaks into very thin strips and season with the black pepper and salt.

4. Melt half the ghee in a large pan over medium-high heat. When the oil becomes hot, fry the steak strips until they turn brown. When all the strips have been fried, set them aside in a bowl.
5. Use the remaining ghee to sauté the onions and garlic for about two minutes. Then add the mushroom slices. Cook for three minutes and stir occasionally.
6. Pour the paprika and mustard into the pan, followed by the bone broth and lemon juice. Bring the mixture to a boil before adding the slices of beef and sour cream.
7. Remove the pan from the heat.
8. Serve with Keto bread focaccia (see recipe in breakfast section)

Nutritional Values Per Serving:
- Calories – 520
- Fat – 38.4 g
- Protein – 34.9 g
- Net carbs – 8.4 g
- Fiber – 1.4 g

Keto Beef Burgundy

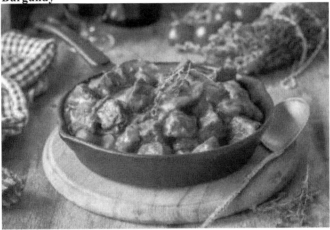

Yield: 6 servings
Ingredients:
2 lbs beef braising steaks
8.5 oz bacon, sliced
3 tbsp ghee
4 cups sliced mushrooms
3 cloves garlic, minced
1 tbsp unsweetened tomato paste
1 white onion, diced
1 large carrot, sliced
Bottle of 750 ml Burgundy
Salt, to taste
For The Bouquet Garni:

3 bay leaves
3 cloves
2 sprigs parsley
1 tsp peppercorn
2 sprigs thyme

Method:

1. Slice the steak into chunks and use salt to season.
2. Melt the ghee in a heavy pot over medium-high heat and fry the steak chunks. When they turn golden-brown on one side, flip over and cook the other side for three minutes. Cook in batches to avoid overcrowding the pot.
3. When ready, set the beef chunks aside in a bowl.
4. Reduce heat to low and cook the onions, sliced carrots, and garlic. Add the beef chunks and tomato paste. Pour in some red wine, enough to almost cover all the meat. Mix well using a spatula and bring to a boil.
5. To make the bouquet garni, take a piece of cheesecloth and place all the herbs in it. Tie the cloth with kitchen twine and place in the pot. Cover the pot and cook for three hours.
6. Once the beef becomes tender, remove the pot from the heat. Scoop out the bouquet garni and cover the pot.
7. In another pan, melt the leftover ghee and cook the bacon slices for five minutes. Then add the sliced mushrooms and cook for five more minutes.
8. When the bacon and mushrooms have turned brown, pour them into the pot of beef. Mix well.
9. Serve and enjoy!

Nutritional Values Per Serving:

- Calories – 678
- Fat – 45 g
- Protein – 36.7 g
- Net carbs – 6.9 g
- Fiber – 1.3 g

Beef Steak With Mustard Sauce

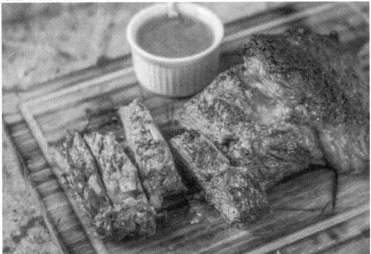

Yield: 2 servings
Ingredients:
For The Steak:
14.1 oz filet mignon steaks
1 tbsp ghee
Salt and pepper, to taste
For The Mustard Sauce:
1 tbsp Dijon mustard
1 tbsp ghee
¼ cup chicken stock
¼ cup coconut milk
½ small onion, diced
½ tsp salt
Method:
1. Use the salt and pepper to generously season the steak.
2. Place a pan over medium heat and melt the ghee. Cook the steaks until they turn brown and then set them aside on a wire rack, covered with foil.
3. Using the same pan, melt the ghee over medium-high heat and add the onions, coconut milk, bone broth, and mustard. Lower heat to medium and bring to a boil.
4. Cook the sauce until it turns creamy.
5. Slice the steak into strips and serve with the mustard sauce.

Nutritional Values Per Serving:
- Calories – 775
- Fat – 65.2 g
- Protein – 39.5 g
- Net carbs – 3.3 g

- Fiber – 1.4 g

Rutabaga Gratin

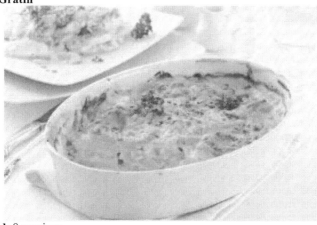

Yield: 8 servings
Ingredients:
8 slices bacon
2.2 lb rutabaga
1 cup cheddar cheese, grated
3 tbsp ghee
1 medium white onion
3 cups vegetable or chicken stock
1 tbsp fresh thyme, chopped
1 cup heavy cream
Black pepper and salt, to taste
For The Topping:
½ cup parmesan cheese, grated
½ cup sour cream
Chopped parsley
Method:
1. Preheat the oven to 320 degrees F.
2. Place a pan over medium heat and melt the ghee. Sauté the chopped onions for about four minutes.
3. Cut the bacon into pieces and fry in the pan. Add thyme and fry until the bacon turns light brown. Remove the pan and set it aside.
4. Peel and then boil the rutabaga in water for 10 minutes. Drain the water and then cut ⅛-inch slices.
5. Grease a large baking tray with ghee and arrange the first layer of rutabaga slices. Add half of the fried bacon and onions and top with grated cheese. Add the second layer of rutabaga and repeat the process. Finally, finish up with the final layer of rutabaga.
6. Pour the vegetable stock, heavy cream, salt, and pepper into a bowl. Mix well and then pour over the rutabaga. It should almost cover the top layer of slices. Add more salt and pepper if you prefer.

7. Cover with foil and place in the oven. Bake for 60 minutes until the rutabaga becomes soft. Open the foil and use a spatula to push the rutabaga slices down into the liquid. Bake for one more hour.
8. When ready, remove the baking tray and set aside.
9. Raise the oven temperature to 400 degrees F.
10. Top the rutabaga mixture with the grated parmesan and sour cream. Put the baking tray back into the oven and bake for 30 minutes to melt the cheese and turn the top layer crispy.
11. Remove and garnish with parsley.
12. Serve with meat or crispy greens.

Nutritional Values Per Serving:
- Calories – 445
- Fat – 37.7 g
- Protein – 13.9 g
- Net carbs – 10.2 g
- Fiber – 3 g

Hot 'N' Creamy Chicken Paprika

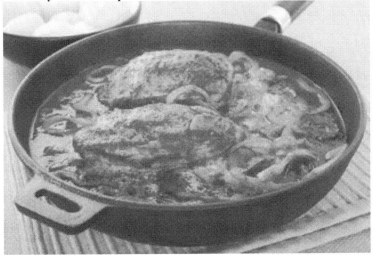

Yield: 4 servings
Ingredients:
8 chicken breasts
1 cup chicken stock
1 medium red pepper
1 medium onion
1 tbsp paprika
2 large tomatoes
2 large green capsicums
¼ cup sour cream
2 tbsp ghee
¼ cup coconut milk

Black pepper and salt, to taste
Method:
1. Use paper towels to pat the chicken breasts dry. Then use salt and black pepper to season.
2. Melt a little ghee in a large soup pot. When hot, cook the chicken over medium-high heat.
3. When the chicken turns brown all over, add the chicken stock and bring to boil. Cover the pot, reduce heat, and cook for 30 minutes. Remove the chicken using tongs and set aside.
4. Chop the onion, capsicums, and tomatoes. Cut the red pepper in half and remove the seeds before you slice it.
5. Sauté the onion using the leftover ghee until brown and then add the capsicums, tomatoes, and red pepper. Cook for another five minutes.
6. Pour the onion mixture into the pot containing chicken stock. Add the paprika and stir. Remove the pot from the heat.
7. Mix the sauce using a hand blender until smooth. Return the pot back to low heat and add the coconut milk and sour cream.
8. Add the chicken breasts back into the pot and cook for five minutes.
9. Serve with cauliflower rice.

Nutritional Value Per Serving:
- Calories – 669
- Fat – 60.7 g
- Protein – 23.7 g
- Net carbs – 4.4 g
- Fiber – 1.7 g

Keto Quiche Lorraine

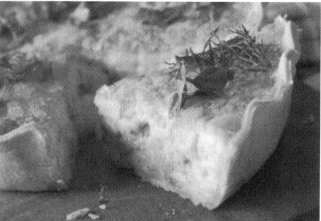

Yield: 10 servings
Ingredients:
For The Base:
2 oz melted butter
1 egg

2 pinches white pepper
A pinch of salt
2 cups almond meal
For The Filling:
5 oz Gruyere cheese
½ brown onion, diced
4 slices bacon
1 tsp Dijon mustard
3 eggs
A pinch of salt
1 ½ cups whipping cream
2 pinches white pepper
Method:
1. Preheat the oven to 340 degrees F.
2. Combine the almond meal, pepper, salt, egg, and melted butter.
3. Pour the mixture into a quiche dish, press it down, and spread it uniformly around the bottom and sides of the dish.
4. Bake for 10 minutes. In case the base starts to rise, burst the air bubble using a fork and press it back down. When ready, remove the base from the oven.
5. To make the filling, place a non-stick pan over medium heat and sauté the bacon. Chop the onions and add to the bacon.
6. When the onions become translucent, pour the mixture into the quiche dish and grate the Gruyere cheese over the quiche. Ensure an even spread over the quiche.
7. Combine the cream, white pepper, salt, eggs, and mustard in a mixing bowl. Use a stick blender to mix the ingredients.
8. Pour the creamy mixture into the quiche dish and return the quiche to the oven. Bake for 30 minutes. When the middle of the quiche turns slightly hard, it is ready.
9. Slice the quiche into 10 wedges and serve.

Nutritional Values Per Serving:
- Calories – 519
- Fat – 46 g
- Protein – 16 g
- Net carbs – 8.8 g
- Fiber – 5 g

Keto Oxtail Stew

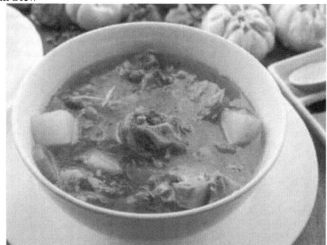

Yield: 8 servings
Ingredients:
3.5 lbs oxtails
1 sprig thyme
2 sprigs rosemary
2 celery stalks, sliced
2 cups green beans, chopped
1 medium rutabaga, diced
¼ cup ghee
3 bay leaves
2 medium leeks, sliced
2 tbsp lemon juice
14.1 oz tin of unsweetened tomatoes
¼ tsp ground cloves
2 quarts water
Salt and pepper, to taste

Method:
1. Pat the oxtails dry using paper towels and season with salt and pepper.
2. Place a large pot over medium-high heat and melt the ghee. Cook the oxtails for 10 minutes until they turn brown.
3. Add the bay leaves, cloves, thyme and rosemary. Pour in the water and lemon juice and bring to a boil. Reduce heat to low and cover the pot. Simmer for three hours until the meat softens.
4. When ready, lift the meat out of the pot using kitchen tongs and set aside. After the oxtail cools, shred the meat from the bones.
5. Peel the rutabaga and dice it before tossing the pieces into the pot. Cover the pot and cook for 10 minutes. Then add the sliced leeks, green beans, tomatoes, and celery stalks. Cook until the rutabaga becomes soft.

6. Return the shredded oxtail meat into the pot and season with salt and pepper.
7. Serve and enjoy!

Nutritional Values Per Serving:
- Calories – 371
- Fat – 21.5 g
- Protein – 32.6 g
- Net carbs – 8.2 g
- Fiber – 2.7 g

Autumn Harvest Stew

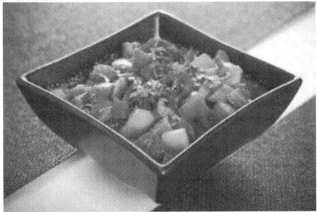

Yield: 10 servings
Ingredients:
10 beef braising steaks, boneless (5.3 oz each)
4 cloves garlic
2 cinnamon sticks
2 bay leaves
1 white onion
2.2 lb zucchini
1.3 lb rutabaga
14.1 oz tin of chopped tomatoes
½ cup lard
1 cup water
1 tsp ground ginger
1 tsp coriander seeds
1 tsp turmeric powder
1 tsp chili powder
2 tbsp paprika
2 tbsp ground cumin
Salt and black pepper, to taste
Method:
1. Preheat a large crockpot on high heat. Use a paper towel to dry the steaks and season all sides with salt and pepper.

2. Melt ¼ cup of lard in a pan and cook the steaks in twos or threes. Cover the pan until the meat turns light brown.
3. Remove the steaks and place them in the preheated crockpot.
4. Meanwhile dice the garlic and onions. Grease a pan with the remaining lard and cook the diced herbs. When they turn light brown, add the tomatoes and all the spices and herbs. Mix for a minute and pour into the crockpot.
5. Add the bay leaves and cinnamon sticks and cover the crockpot. Cook for three hours. In the meantime, dice the rutabaga and zucchini.
6. After the steak has cooked for three hours, move the meat to one side of the pot using a spatula. Add the rutabaga on the other side. Cook for one hour and then add the zucchini on the rutabaga side. Submerge the rutabaga and zucchini in the stew and cook for two hours.
7. When the rutabaga and zucchini become soft, turn off the heat.
8. Serve garnished with cilantro and seasoned with salt and pepper.

Nutritional Values Per Serving:
- Calories – 533
- Fat – 39.5 g
- Protein – 31.9 g
- Net carbs – 9.1 g
- Fiber – 3.6 g

Chorizo Stuffed Zucchini

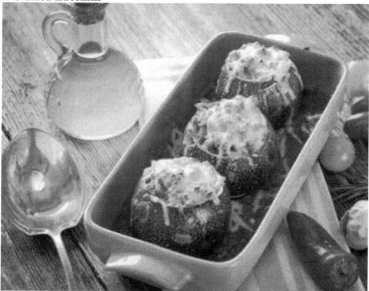

Yield: 4 servings
Ingredients:
4 medium round zucchinis
1 ½ cups chanterelle mushrooms
4.2 oz Mexican chorizo

1 cup cheddar cheese, grated
2 tbsp lard/ghee
Salt and pepper, to taste
Method:
1. Preheat the oven to 350 degrees F.
2. Slice the tops off the zucchinis and use a spoon to scoop out the flesh into a bowl. Leave a shell about ½-inch thick.
3. Brush the tops and insides of the zucchinis with melted lard and arrange them on a baking sheet. Place in the oven for 15 minutes.
4. Meanwhile, chop the mushrooms and chorizo.
5. Grease a pan with melted lard and cook the chorizo over medium heat until they turn crispy.
6. Toss in the mushrooms and stir well. Cook for five minutes before adding the flesh of the zucchini. Cook for three more minutes and then set aside.
7. Grate the cheese over the pan and mix with the chorizo, mushrooms, and zucchini flesh. Add seasoning to taste.
8. Scoop the mixture into the zucchini shells and place in the oven for 15 minutes.
9. Serve with crispy greens and enjoy!

Nutritional Values Per Serving:
- Calories – 388
- Fat – 29.8 g
- Protein – 21.7 g
- Net carbs – 7 g
- Fiber – 4.4 g

Egg And Bacon Stuffed Zucchini

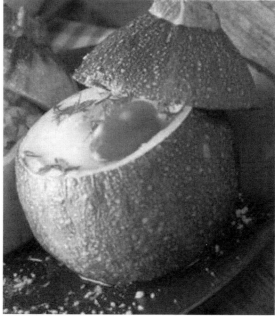

Yield: 4 servings
Ingredients:
4 medium eggs
4 slices bacon, sliced
4 round zucchinis
3 oz parmesan cheese
2 cloves garlic
1.9 oz ghee, melted
1 white onion
Salt and pepper, to taste
Method:
1. Preheat the oven to 350 degrees F.
2. Slice the top of the zucchinis off, scoop out the flesh with a spoon, and set the flesh aside.
3. Brush the insides of the zucchinis with melted ghee and arrange them on a baking sheet. Place in the oven for 20 minutes.
4. Meanwhile, chop the onion and garlic.
5. Grease a pan with melted ghee and cook the onion and garlic over medium heat. Then toss in the sliced bacon and cook for 5 minutes until crisp. Stir occasionally.
6. Add the flesh of the zucchini, mix well, and cook for five more minutes. Then set aside. Grate the cheese into the pan and mix well before seasoning with salt and pepper.

7. Scoop the mixture, pour into the shells of the zucchini, and crack an egg inside every shell. Place in the oven for 20 minutes and wait for the egg white to become opaque. The yolk should stay runny.
8. Serve with crispy greens and enjoy!

Nutritional Values Per Serving:
- Calories – 400
- Protein – 19.9 g
- Fat – 31.4 g
- Net carbs – 8 g
- Fiber – 2.7 g

Keto Spinach Omelet

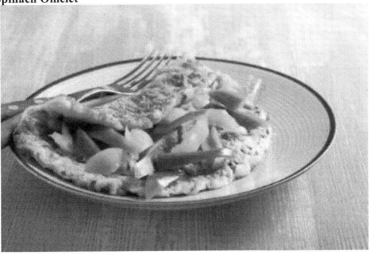

Yield: 1 serving
Ingredients:
3 large eggs
1.8 oz feta cheese, crumbled
1.1 oz ghee
3.5 oz spinach
1 red bell pepper
1 yellow bell pepper
Salt and pepper, to taste
Method:
1. Grease a pan with one tablespoon of ghee. Slice the garlic and cook over medium-high heat. Add salt and cook for one minute.
2. Cook the spinach leaves in the pan for two minutes and then pour the spinach and garlic into a bowl.
3. Take a small bowl and crack the eggs into it. Beat with a fork and add the spinach and crumbled feta. Season with salt and pepper.
4. Grease the pan with the remaining ghee and cook the mixture over medium heat. Move the egg mixture toward the middle of the pan using

a spatula for 30 seconds. Reduce heat and cook for one minute. Take your time when cooking to produce a fluffy and soft omelet.

5. Slice the green and yellow bell peppers and use as topping on the omelet.
6. Fold up the omelet and cook for one minute to warm the peppers.
7. Serve and enjoy!

Nutritional Values Per Serving:

- Calories – 659
- Fat – 55.5 g
- Protein – 30.9 g
- Net carbs – 7
- Fiber – 2.8 g

Watercress Bisque

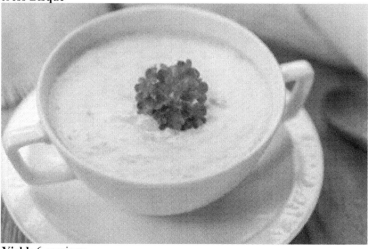

Yield: 6 servings
Ingredients:
5.3 oz watercress
14.1 oz cauliflower
7.1 oz fresh spinach
3.9 oz white onion
1 bay leaf, crumbled
2 cloves garlic
1 cup coconut milk
1/ cup coconut oil
4 cups chicken stock
Salt and ground black pepper, to taste

Method:

1. Dice the garlic and onion.
2. Place a soup pot over medium-high heat and grease with coconut oil. Sauté until onions turn light brown.
3. Wash the watercress and spinach. Chop the cauliflower into florets and cook with the onions. Add the bay leaf and cook for five minutes, stirring frequently.
4. Add watercress and spinach and cook until vegetables wilt.
5. Add chicken stock and bring to boil. When cauliflower becomes soft, add coconut milk.
6. Add salt and black pepper, to taste. Remove pan from heat and pulse with hand blender to create creamy consistency.
7. Serve immediately.

Nutritional Values Per Serving:

- Calories – 392
- Fat – 37.6 g
- Protein – 4.9 g
- Net carbs – 6.8 g
- Fiber – 2.9 g

Eggplant Lasagna

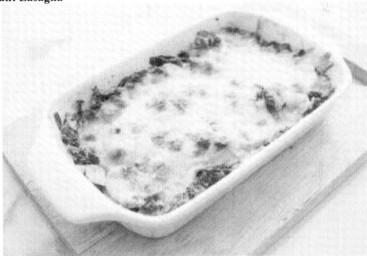

Yield: 6 servings
Ingredients:
1.6 lb eggplants
10.6 oz fresh spinach
6 large eggs
1 cup marinara sauce
1.1 oz parmesan cheese, grated
4 oz mozzarella cheese, grated
7.1 oz feta cheese, crumbled

3 oz ghee
Salt, to taste

Method:

1. Preheat the oven to 400 degrees F.
2. Cut the eggplant into slices ½ inch thick. Melt the ghee and use ¼ of it to grease the slices. Season with salt and cook in the oven for 20 minutes.
3. Boil water in a pot and add spinach leaves. After boiling for one minute, use tongs to immediately dip the boiled leaves in ice cold water. Remove the spinach and drain excess water by squeezing the leaves in a strainer.
4. Remove the baked eggplant from the oven and reduce the temperature to 360 degrees F.
5. Crack one egg into a bowl, add salt, and mix well.
6. Grease a pan using the remaining ghee and cook a thin omelet by swirling the pan around. Set on a plate and do the same for the remaining five eggs.
7. Place two omelets at the bottom of a baking dish. Spread ⅓ of the marinara sauce over the omelet, add ⅓ of the eggplant slices, ⅓ of grated mozzarella, ½ of spinach, ½ of feta cheese, and top with two omelets.
8. Repeat the same process to create another layer of sauce, eggplant, mozzarella, spinach, feta, and omelet. The final layer should be topped with all the parmesan.
9. Place the baking dish in the oven and bake for 30 minutes. Remove when the top becomes golden-brown and let it cool.
10. Slice into six pieces and serve warm or cold.

Nutritional Values Per Serving:

- Calories – 474
- Fat – 38 g
- Protein – 20.8 g
- Net carbs – 8.7 g
- Fiber – 5.4 g

Chorizo Tex Mex Stew

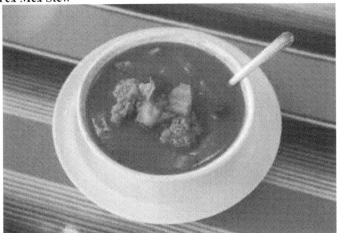

Yield: 8 servings
Ingredients:
7.1 oz chorizo
17.6 oz ground beef
2 cups green beans (optional)
14.1 oz unsweetened tomatoes
2.2 oz unsweetened tomato puree
2 cloves garlic
2 medium tomatoes
1 liter water
2 small green chilis
¼ cup ghee
1 medium red bell pepper
Tabasco, to taste
Salt and black pepper, to taste
Method:
1. Chop the onions and garlic. Then cut the bell and chili peppers in half, remove seeds, and slice them.
2. Place a large pot over medium-high heat, melt the ghee, and sauté the onions and garlic. Stir until onions turn light brown and add the sliced peppers. Cook for five minutes while stirring occasionally.
3. Cut the chorizo into slices and chop the tomatoes into chunks.
4. Add the ground beef and chorizo into the pot and cook until brown. Add all the tomatoes, including the puree, and the Tabasco sauce.
5. Add the water, salt, and black pepper. Chop the green beans and add them to the pot when the soup starts bubbling. Cook for 10 minutes.
6. When green beans become tender, remove the pot from the heat.
7. Serve hot with Keto bread.
Nutritional Values Per Serving:
- Calories – 371

- Fat – 29.2 g
- Protein – 18.4 g
- Net carbs – 6.4 g
- Fiber – 2.2 g

Red Gazpacho With Cream

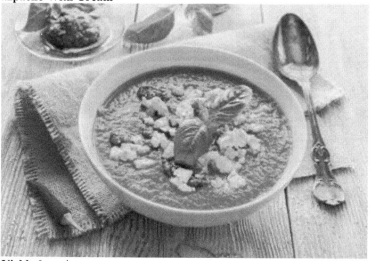

Yield: 6 servings
Ingredients:
14.1 oz tomatoes
1 large cucumber
1 large red pepper
1 large green pepper
2 medium avocados
2 cloves garlic
1 small red onion
1 medium spring onion
2 tbsp basil, chopped
2 tbsp parsley, chopped
1 cup extra virgin olive oil
2 tbsp wine vinegar
2 tbsp lemon juice
7.1 oz feta cheese
Salt and black pepper, to taste
Method:
1. Preheat the oven to 400 degrees F.
2. Slice the bell peppers and take out the seeds. Lay them on a lined baking tray and bake in the oven for 20 minutes.
3. Chop the onion and place in a blender. Cut the avocados, remove the seed from each, and scoop the flesh into the blender. Quarter the tomatoes and toss into the blender.

4. Once the bell peppers are baked, allow them to cool, then peel off the skin and place in the blender.
5. Pour the olive oil, salt, pepper, vinegar, lemon juice, garlic, and fresh herbs into the blender. Mix the ingredients to create smooth puree.
6. Chop the spring onions and cucumber and add to the puree. Blend well.
7. Top with feta cheese and herbs and serve.

Nutritional Values Per Serving:
- Calories – 528
- Fat – 50.8 g
- Protein – 7.5 g
- Net carbs – 8.5 g
- Fiber – 5.8 g

Cauliflower Avgolemono (Greek Soup)

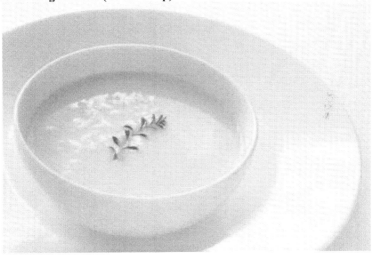

Yield: 8 servings
Ingredients:
14.8 oz cauliflower rice (homemade or prepared from grocery)
1 onion
3 eggs
6 cups chicken broth
17.6 oz chicken breasts, shredded
2 lemons, juiced
½ cup heavy cream
2 cups water
Chopped parsley
Salt and pepper, to taste

Method:
1. Rice the cauliflower by chopping into florets and grating the florets using a box grater.

2. Shred the chicken by first cooking it in a pan and then using two forks to rip the meat apart.
3. Heat a large pot and grease with cooking oil. Sauté the chopped onions until they brown. Then pour in the water, broth, cream, cauliflower rice, and chicken.
4. Add the herbs and lemon juice. Taste to check the flavor.
5. Cook for eight minutes, or until the cauliflower softens.
6. Meanwhile, crack the eggs in a bowl. As you whisk the eggs, pour in a ladle of the hot soup from the pot.
7. Turn off the heat and pour the egg mixture into the pot as you stir.
8. Allow the hot soup to cook the eggs for three minutes.
9. Serve topped with parsley or dill.

Nutritional Values Per Serving:
- Calories – 251
- Fat – 16.3 g
- Protein – 20.7 g
- Net carbs – 6 g
- Fiber – 1.4 g

Thai Fried Noodles And Prawns

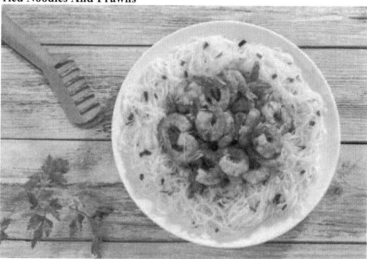

Yield: 4 servings
Ingredients:
2 packs shirataki noodles
2 lbs prawns
6 oz mushrooms, chopped
1/2 red pepper
1 green pepper
¼ c. spring onion
2 cloves garlic
½ c. bean sprouts

1 small chili pepper
3 tbsp fish sauce
1 tbsp ginger, finely chopped
1 tbsp lime juice
 1 tbsp coconut aminos
1 bunch cilantro
Salt, to taste
½ cup extra virgin olive oil

Method:

1. Wash the noodles, boil them, and then fry them in a pan. Set them aside in a bowl.
2. Slice the chili pepper and remove the seeds. Chop off the cilantro stalks and cut them into small pieces. The leaves will be used as garnish. Peel and chop the garlic and ginger, then cut the mushrooms into slices.
3. Place a pan over medium-high heat, grease with olive oil, and fry the cilantro stalks, garlic, chili pepper, and ginger.
4. Peel the raw prawns and fry in the pan until they turn pink. Set the prawns aside. Slice and wash the spring onion. Cut the red and green peppers in half, remove the seeds, and slice into strips.
5. Grease the pan with olive oil and cook the spring onions over medium-high heat for one minute. Add the mushrooms and peppers and cook for two minutes. Then toss in the bean sprouts, stir, and cook for one minute.
6. Pour in the fish sauce, coconut aminos and noodles. Stir well and cook for one minute. Pour in the lime juice and garnish with cilantro leaves.
7. Serve and enjoy!

Nutritional Values Per Serving:

- Calories – 381
- Fat – 29 g
- Protein – 21.5 g
- Net carbs – 8.4 g
- Fiber – 4 g

Creamy Spinach And Salmon

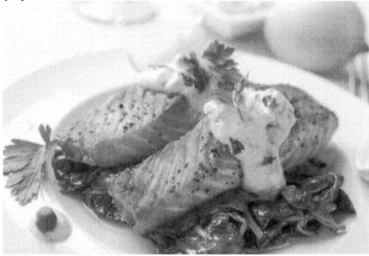

Yield: 1 serving
Ingredients:
4.4 oz fresh spinach
4.4 oz salmon fillet
2 tbsp extra virgin olive oil
1 tbsp coconut milk
Hollandaise sauce
Salt and black pepper, to taste
Method:
1. Preheat oven to 400 degrees F.
2. Put the fillet on a baking tray and sprinkle one tablespoon of olive oil over the fish. Add salt and black pepper.
3. Bake the fish for 20 minutes.
4. Wash the spinach and pat dry using a paper towel.
5. Place a skillet over medium heat and use the remaining olive oil to cook the spinach for four minutes. Add salt, to taste.
6. Pour the coconut milk over the spinach and then remove the pan from the heat.
7. When the fillet is ready, remove it from the oven.
8. Serve the spinach on a plate and place the fillet on top.
9. Pour the Hollandaise sauce over the fillet.
10. Enjoy!
Nutritional Values Per Serving:
- Calories – 813
- Fat – 72.6 g
- Protein – 34 g
- Net carbs – 3.7 g
- Fiber – 2.8 g

Closing Remarks

Thanks for sticking with me to the end of this book!

By now, I hope you understand what a keto cleanse is and all the benefits you stand to gain from following a keto diet. I have also provided you with a 28-day meal plan that you can easily follow for the duration of your 28-day keto cleanse, complete with the recipes for these delicious, easy, and low-carb meals. The recipes contained in this book will help you keep your carbs low and maintain a healthy lifestyle that will keep you energized and keep diseases at bay.

All you need to do now it to commit to getting started on your keto cleanse. Good luck on your keto journey!

About the Author:

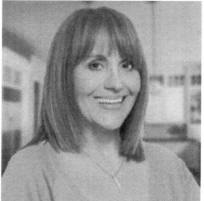

Andrea Adams apart from being an author, is an entrepreneur, activist and proud wife and mother. After quitting her corporate job at a prestigious marketing firm in Denver 5 years ago, she started a health food café with her sister, Marta. The café was a great success and has since opened several other locations in Colorado. Andrea only works part-time in managing the business and has taken a step back to focus on her real passion: creating recipes and writing.

When she is not experimenting in the kitchen, you'll find her hiding in a quiet corner of the house plugging away on her laptop—that is, when she is not cheering in the stands at her sons' football games or helping them with their homework. She also fosters stray dogs and helped found a shelter for injured and abused animals. She now lives in Boulder with her husband and three sons.

40618073R00059

Made in the USA
Lexington, KY
31 May 2019